THE BEST

PRESSURE COOKER

RECIPES

CINDA CHAVICH

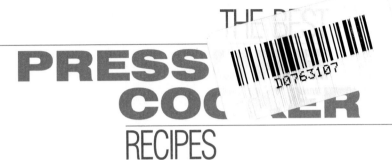

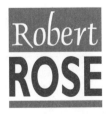

Robert
ROSE

The Best Pressure Cooker Recipes

Copyright © 2001 Cinda Chavich

For complete cataloguing information, see page 4.

DESIGN, EDITORIAL AND PRODUCTION:	MATTHEWS COMMUNICATIONS DESIGN INC.
PHOTOGRAPHY:	MARK T. SHAPIRO
ART DIRECTION/FOOD PHOTOGRAPHY:	SHARON MATTHEWS
FOOD STYLIST:	KATE BUSH
PROP STYLIST:	CHARLENE ERRICSON
RECIPE EDITORS/TEST KITCHEN:	LESLEIGH LANDRY/JENNIFER MACKENZIE
MANAGING EDITOR:	PETER MATTHEWS
INDEXER:	BARBARA SCHON
COLOR SCANS:	POINTONE GRAPHICS

We acknowledge the financial support of the Government of Canada through the Book Publishing Industry Development Program (BPIDP) for our publishing activities.

Published by: Robert Rose Inc. • 120 Eglinton Ave. E., Suite 1000
Toronto, Ontario, Canada M4P 1E2   Tel: (416) 322-6552

Printed in Canada

1234567 BP 04 03 02 01

Contents

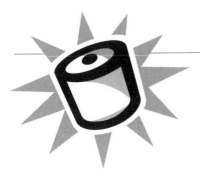

National Library of Canada Cataloguing in Publication Data

In the U.S.A.

Chavich, Cinda
   The best pressure cooker recipes

1st ed.
For use in the United States.
Includes index.
ISBN 0-7788-0028-8

1. Pressure cookery.   I. Title.

TX840.P7C42 2001a   641.5'87   C2001-930017-4

In Canada

Chavich, Cinda
   The best pressure cooker recipes

1st ed.
For use in Canada.
Includes index.
ISBN 0-7788-0031-8

1. Pressure cookery.   I. Title.

TX840.P7C42 2001   641.5'87   C2001-930007-7

Introduction

WHEN IT COMES TO NAMING THE KITCHEN TOOL of the millennium, I cast my vote for today's new generation of pressure cooker.

As a professional food writer, I have purchased almost every gadget and gizmo for my well-stocked kitchen. Some are the kinds that do the job nicely when you need them (which may be rarely). Some, like the microwave, are inadequate for cooking most things from scratch, but are invaluable for defrosting, steaming, melting and reheating. Others I have relegated to the culinary scrap heap – they just don't deliver acceptable results.

For many years, I had put pressure cookers in the latter category. Not that they didn't work. But the old 1950s-style cookers *were* a little frightening. Like most people, I had heard of some nasty disaster that occurred when a pressure cooker blew a gasket. And who needed to risk life and limb – never mind the prospect of mopping up a steam-propelled eruption of food – just to cook dinner a little faster?

Then I began to notice that pressure cookers were starting to appear in all the best kitchen stores. These fancy new models were reportedly foolproof. And while I was skeptical, professional curiosity got the better of me. Eventually I broke down and set out to purchase one of these sexy new devices.

Looking at the new models available, it quickly became clear that these were not the same pressure cookers of a generation ago. Sleek and shiny, most were heavy-bottomed, stainless steel pots – ranging in size from that of a deep sauté pan to a large stockpot – with loads of safety devices.

Gone is the hissing, jiggly pressure regulator that always seemed unreliable at best. In its place, most modern machines have a new pressure regulator and quick-release valve, which allows you to release the steam from the pot without hauling the hot and heavy monster over to the cold water tap to cool it down.

With many of the new cookers, you are now unable to build pressure unless the lid is properly affixed; similarly, it is almost impossible to inadvertently clog the main pressure vent – and end up with lima beans all over your walls.

Still, the safety and convenience of today's new pressure cookers isn't what hooked me. It was the food.

Hands-free risotto, cooked to creamy perfection in 6 minutes. The house filled with the heady aromas of tender beef and red wine stew in half an hour. Almost-instant homemade stocks and broths, with all of the infused flavor you'd expect from hours of slow cooking.

This is what has really made the pressure cooker indispensable in my kitchen. You can't cook everything in a pressure cooker but, like a food processor, it's a tool that can save you time and energy without compromising quality.

Like many people, I am trying to eat more healthy, homemade and unprocessed foods. That means more vegetarian meals, beans and whole grains. I also want to serve more international dishes – Indian curries, Mexican black bean soups, French cassoulet and saffron-infused Spanish stews. The problem is that no one has the extra time typically required to cook these meals, especially on a busy weekday.

That's where the pressure cooker really shines. Dishes that used to take hours are now ready in just a fraction of that time. You can expect to cook a soup or stew in one-third the time (or less) when compared with a conventional recipe. Dried beans are ready to eat in anywhere from 4 to 15 minutes. Hulled barley or wheat berries are tender in less than 45 minutes.

The cooker can also save you money and culinary boredom. Now you have time to do more than the standard chicken breasts and pork cutlets: In the same time it takes to grill or sauté an expensive cut, you can have succulent short ribs, tender chicken stew or a healthy bean dish. So think about savory stew, coq au vin, or rogan josh tonight. Have a healthy grain pilaf with your grilled chicken or simmer a big pot of bean soup for lunch in less than 15 minutes. Once you serve a pot roast that tastes and smells like it's been simmering all day, you'll be hooked – guaranteed.

Unlike many of the "fad" kitchen appliances that come and go, your new pressure cooker will be one that you'll never regret buying. In fact, if you're like me, you won't know what you did without it!

The essentials of pressure cooking

The theory of pressure cooking is simple. By subjecting a sealed pot to heat, pressure builds up inside the unit. This pressure – typically maintained at between 5 and 15 pounds per square inch (psi) – causes the food inside to be cooked at about 250° F (120° C), some 38° F (20° C) hotter than the normal boiling point. The result is that cooking times are significantly reduced. Most foods will cook in one-third the time of conventional boiling or braising.

THE EVOLUTION OF THE PRESSURE COOKER

It was a French inventor in the 17th century who first screwed a lid firmly onto a cast iron pot to trap steam. He discovered that the steam increased the cooking temperature 15 percent above the normal boiling point. Nearly 200 years later, another inventive Frenchman perfected a method of preserving food under high pressure and the seeds of home pressure cooking were sown.

Huge home pressure canners were introduced in North America by National Presto Industries in 1915 and, by the 1940s, many manufacturers were selling "pressure saucepans" to busy homemakers.

The early pressure cookers were very straightforward devices, consisting of a heavy pot and lid that was locked on top. The seal was provided by a rubber gasket and the pressure was controlled by a heavy weight that sat loosely on top of a vent pipe in the lid. As steam built up inside the cooker, the pressure would lift the weight slightly, allowing steam to escape. This cycle of pressure build-up and release caused the weight to jiggle and hiss continuously throughout the cooking time – hence the term "jiggle-top" used to describe these old-fashioned cookers.

While the jiggle-top cookers were functional, they also presented some risks. If the steam vent became clogged, the pressure could build to dangerous levels, requiring the cook to place the pot immediately under cold running water to avoid blowing the emergency release plug – and sending food all over the kitchen.

By the 1970s, the popularity of pressure cookers had declined in North America, and the microwave oven became the preferred way to cook food quickly. But Europeans rejected this new kind of cooking. And over the next 25 years, European manufacturers like Italy's Lagostina, France's T-Fal and Switzerland's Kuhn-Rikon worked to perfect the home pressure cooker with innovations that made them easy and safe to use. Today, while most European households use pressure cookers to prepare food quickly, North Americans are only just beginning to rediscover the benefits of these devices.

The latest generation of pressure cookers feature a stationary pressure regulator, either a fixed weight or spring valve. This system keeps the pressure even by occasionally releasing a burst of steam, and allows the cook to quickly release the pressure in the cooker at the end of the cooking time by pressing a button or flipping a switch. This type of system is less likely to clog than the old weight-valve mechanism which, because it emits steam constantly, has a much greater chance of getting a piece of food stuck in the vent pipe.

The new cookers also have backup release mechanisms so that it's impossible to have a pressure cooker explosion. While older models were designed with a steam valve or plug that would blow out if excess pressure built up inside the unit (spewing the contents over the kitchen), this isn't possible with the new generation of pressure cookers.

Most have several preventative safety features. When the cooker comes up to pressure, a lid-locking mechanism pops up. This tells you that the unit has reached full pressure and prevents you from opening the lid when the contents are under pressure.

Many cookers also have one or two secondary safety valves – usually on the lid and around the gasket – which are designed to emit steam (not contents) if the main pressure valve malfunctions or becomes clogged with food during cooking.

What to look for in a pressure cooker

The most important thing to remember when buying a pressure cooker is that, as in all things, you get what you pay for. Decide before you shop what is important to you.

The pricier cookers have more bells and whistles, more safety features and heavier bottoms. If you're perfectly comfortable dealing with the jiggle-top technology of bygone years, there are lots of inexpensive pressure cookers available in this category. But if you need a boost to get past the fear of pressure cooking, choose one of the second-generation cookers.

Look for a cooker with a lock that makes the lid impossible to remove when there is any pressure still inside. Find out what kind of backup valve there is to release pressure if the main valve becomes clogged. In older and less-sophisticated models, the valve is simply a rubber plug that will blow out and launch the contents of the cooker into your kitchen. The latest models offer one or more pressure releases that will vent the steam, not the contents, if there is a malfunction in the main pressure valve.

Do your homework (most cooker manufacturers have Internet sites that describe their products). Check out the offerings of as many stores as possible. A number of the new-generation cookers from companies like Lagostina, T-Fal, Kuhn-Rikon and Presto, are still only sold in specialty kitchen stores or high-end boutiques.

Try opening and closing the pressure cooker. Is it easy to lock the lid in place? Would you feel comfortable opening the cooker when it's extremely hot? Imagine lifting the pressure cooker when it's hot and full of soup or stew. Are the handles comfortable? Will they stay cool?

Look at the pressure release valve. Some release a jet of steam straight into the air, others shoot it out at an angle (saving your ceiling from a moisture bath). If there are two settings or a dial, you can release the steam gradually. Some cookers simply have a metal bale to flip – the steam comes out quickly in all directions and the bale can be very hot. Others require that you push the valve down with your finger (or a wooden spoon) to release the steam – fairly simple, but still time-consuming, since you can't just walk away while the pressure drops.

If you buy a less sophisticated model (without a spring-loaded pressure release valve) you will have to remove the pan from the heat and allow the pressure to reduce naturally, or pick up the hot pressure cooker, take it to the sink and run it under cold water until the heat and steam dissipates.

Do you plan to steam desserts in your cooker? If so, you'll want a model that offers at least two pressure settings – high (13 to 15 psi) and low (5 to 8 psi) – because most cakes and steamed puddings don't rise well when cooked at high pressure. Low pressure is also useful for delicate foods and thick sauces that tend to burn easily.

Choose a cooker that's large enough to accommodate whole roasts – a 6- or 7-litre model is good for most families. A small, skillet-style cooker is good for vegetables and delicate foods that you want to bring to pressure and steam very quickly.

A pressure cooker with a larger cooking surface and good, heavy base will make browning easier and burning less likely. A quality stainless steel surface is easy to clean. Some companies offer pressure cookware sets, with both deep and shallow pans that will accommodate the same pressure lid, as well as regular glass lids so that you can also use the pans for conventional cooking.

WHAT FOOD IS BEST PREPARED IN A PRESSURE COOKER?

While the pressure cooker is a wonderfully versatile appliance, it is better for some types of food than others. For example, it is ideal for just about any comfort food – soups, tender stews, pot roasts and creamy risottos. Not only does it give you perfect results, you can cut the usual cooking time down by two-thirds.

Beans, tougher cuts of meat, soups, stews, chilies and grains are also perfect candidates for your pressure cooker.

And don't forget desserts. You will never bake a cheesecake again after you've tried the smooth, creamy versions you can create in your pressure cooker. It also makes wonderful rice pudding, crème caramel and steamed Christmas pudding in a fraction of the time you're used to.

You can also almost instantly cook tender cuts of chicken (breasts are done in only 8 minutes) and perfectly steam fish in the pressure cooker in 3 minutes flat.

Or you can use the cooker as a tool to prep ingredients – dried chickpeas for hummus, beans and whole grains for healthy salads, and cooked fruits for preserves. Beans can be instantly quick-soaked in the pressure cooker, most varieties in less than a minute.

The pressure cooker is perfect for making rich homemade stocks with recycled soup bones and vegetable scraps. Chicken pieces and ribs can be pre-cooked and flavor-infused quickly for finishing on the barbecue. Corn-on-the-cob never touches water when steamed in its own juice on the trivet in less than 2 minutes.

Cooking under high pressure helps to break down the connective tissues in tougher cuts of meat, retains water-soluble nutrients that are normally boiled away, and instantly infuses and mingles flavors in a way that is usually found only in slow-cooked food. And unlike other appliances (like slow cookers), you can brown meats and vegetables in the pan before pressure cooking, adding extra layers of flavor that come from caramelizing sugars.

ADAPTING CONVENTIONAL RECIPES FOR THE PRESSURE COOKER

Almost any recipe that requires long and slow cooking, simmering, braising or steaming can easily be adapted for pressure cooking.

Think of all of your favorite peasant cuisines – from braised Spanish beans and French lamb stews to slow-simmered Indian curries, Asian hot pots, goulash, stroganoff, pot roasts and comforting beef stew. You probably have many favorite family recipes that your mother or grandmother served which could be completed in less than half the traditional time in a pressure cooker.

The high heat and pressure works to instantly tenderize tougher cuts of meat, so you can start to enjoy delicious and inexpensive meals, even when you're pressed for time after work. Try recipes using round steak, short ribs, stewing beef, lamb shanks and turkey parts. You'll be amazed at the intense flavor that these cuts can add to everyday meals.

One of the main differences between conventional and pressure cooking recipes is the amount of liquid required. In the pressure cooker, most stews need less than 2 cups (500 mL) broth, stewed tomatoes, coconut milk or other saucy ingredients. Remember that vegetables and meats will release liquid while cooking, about 1/4 cup (50 mL) for every 2 cups (500 mL) raw veggies.

Plan to thicken your dishes at the end of the cooking process. I have found that a flour *roux* used at the start of my favorite Cajun-style stews and gumbos burned in the intense heat of the pressure cooker. The solution: make the *roux* on the side and whisk it into the stew after the pressure has been released.

Pressure cooking also requires a different approach to using herbs and spices. The high heat of pressure cooking destroys the flavor in delicate herbs, and even the most robust herbs if used fresh. Plan to use dried herbs in your recipes (and in greater quantites), or add your fresh chopped herbs at the end of cooking.

STEPS TO SUCCESSFUL PRESSURE COOKING

Cooking under pressure is easy if you follow a few simple steps.

Browning (where appropriate). While it's not absolutely necessary to brown meats and vegetables before pressure cooking, I heartily recommend it. Most stews, soups and pot roasts benefit greatly from the added flavor that comes with browning and caramelizing sugars before cooking.

Filling. Don't overfill the pressure cooker. Make sure the pot is never more than two-thirds full. If you're cooking beans, rice or grains (which foam up during cooking), make sure the pot is no more than half full. Some cookers have a maximum fill indicator line stamped on the pot. Conversely, be sure you don't *underfill* the cooker. Consult the manufacturer's instruction booklet to determine the minimum amount of liquid required for pressure cooking in your unit, usually at least 1/2 to 1 cup (125 to 250 mL).

If you are steaming food on a rack, place a metal trivet or steaming basket inside the unit, add the water and place the food directly on the rack or in a heatproof plate or casserole dish. The trivet or basket is designed to keep the water level below the food you are cooking – so don't add too much water.

Lock the lid. Make sure the lid is properly closed before putting the pressure cooker on the heat. Some pressure cookers have dots or marks you will need to line up before twisting the lid to lock it. With others, you pull a lever across or push a button to activate the lock.

Bring cooker to full pressure. Get the pressure cooker up to full pressure as quickly as possible by putting it over high heat. If you have a multi-level valve, choose the appropriate "psi" setting. It can take several minutes to achieve full pressure. Use a burner that is no larger than the base of the pot and, if you are cooking with gas, be sure the flame isn't licking up the sides. You can tell when the cooker is up to full pressure in several ways. New models have a button that rises to indicate that pressure has been reached, and will hiss slightly until you reduce the heat. On old jiggle-top models, the weight will begin to jiggle rapidly; reduce the heat immediately or you will have a blow-out.

Reduce heat, just to maintain even pressure. Once the cooker is up to pressure, reduce the heat to low or medium-low. You want to maintain an even pressure during cooking, but you shouldn't hear too much steam escaping (an indication that the heat is too high). With a jiggle-top model, the jiggler should just barely continue to rock, about 4 or 5 times a minute. A fixed weight valve should not sputter but may emit a very soft hissing sound, while a spring-valve cooker will be quite silent, with its valve stem rising to the desired level without dropping.

Watch the cooking time. Begin timing when the unit is up to pressure and use an accurate timer (I used the timer on my microwave) to make sure that you release the pressure as soon as the time is up. If you are pressure cooking at high altitudes, you will have to adjust the cooking times. Add about 5 percent more time for every 1,000 feet (300 m) above sea level. If you find the food is not properly cooked when you remove the lid, lock the lid back in place, bring the pressure cooker back up to full pressure over high heat, reduce heat to low and cook for another 1 or 2 minutes longer. You can also finish the cooking conventionally; this is especially desirable if you want to reduce the cooking liquid to thicken a sauce or stew.

For a convenient list of recommended cooking times for different types of food, see pages 15 to 17.

Release the pressure. When the instructions in a recipe call for releasing the pressure naturally, simply remove the pressure cooker from the heat and wait for the pressure indicator to drop. When the pressure has dissipated, the locking mechanism (on those cookers so equipped) disengages and you can remove the lid. Tilt the lid away from you when opening it. The "natural release" method is best for beans and grains, which can break up and clog the valve if you release the pressure quickly. This method also keeps fragile items like beans intact. It's also good for large pieces of meat (which can toughen), and for soups and stocks, which can spew out when the pressure is released too quickly.

If the recipe calls for releasing the pressure quickly (appropriate for many dishes, and those that might overcook if left under pressure), simply release the pressure valve by pressing the button or flipping the lever. A steady jet of steam will flow out of the machine until all of the pressure has been released. (Be careful, the steam can be hot!) Then the pressure indicator/locking mechanism button will drop and allow you to remove the lid.

If the cooker doesn't have a quick-release valve, you will have to take it to the sink and run cold water over the lid, being careful not to run water into the steam valve, until you hear the locking mechanism release. Some models do not have a locking mechanism to prevent opening the unit while there is still pressure inside. If the lid is removed before all of the pressure has dissipated, the food inside can erupt and burn you. Be careful.

Cleaning the pressure cooker

Read the manufacturer's directions for cleaning your pressure cooker and clean it after every use. Safety devices can fail if the unit is not properly maintained.

Always remove the rubber gasket and clean it with warm soapy water after cooking, then replace it under the rim of the lid. Don't immerse the lid in water or place it in the dishwasher. Remove the jiggle top or spring valve and make sure there is no food clogging the steam vent. You can run water through the vent pipe or use a pipe cleaner to remove any build-up. Look through vent to make sure it's clear every time you close the cover.

Some manufacturers also recommend removing the pressure regulator valve and running it under hot water to clean. Also check the secondary safety valve and clean out any food deposits.

Replace the rubber gasket every year or so. When storing the pressure cooker, store the lid separately or invert it on top to preserve the elasticity of the gasket and eliminate cooking odors.

TROUBLESHOOTING

The best source of information about your pressure cooker is the manufacturer. Read the printed material that comes with the cooker for toll-free help lines and websites.

Always follow the manufacturer's instructions. Each pressure cooker works differently and may have unique requirements.

If the cooker begins to hiss loudly during cooking, immediately remove it from the heat. If either or both of the safety release devices engage, turn off the heat and allow the cooker to cool down before removing the lid. Clean all parts well before starting over.

Never leave the pressure cooker unattended. Never deep-fry in the pressure cooker.

Unless you have a new-generation pressure cooker with extra built-in safety systems, avoid cooking applesauce, cranberries, barley, split peas, rhubarb, pasta or cereals — all of which are infamous for clogging up the works.

SOURCES

If you need more information about pressure cookers, sources include:

Lagostina 1-800-263-4067 www.lagostina.com

Kuhn Rikon 1-800-662-5882 415-461-1048
www.kuhnrikon.com

Mirro Company 1-800-527-7727 www.mirro.com

T-Fal Canada Inc. 416-297-4131 www.t-fal.com

National Presto Industries 1-800-877-0441 www.presto-net.com

Table of cooking times

VEGETABLES	COOKING TIME (APPROX.) *steamed on rack over 1 to 2 cups (250 to 500 mL) boiling water*
Artichoke, medium, trimmed	6 to 8 minutes
Artichokes, small, trimmed	5 to 6 minutes
Asparagus	1 to 2minutes
Beans, green or yellow	2 to 3 minutes
Beets, small, whole	12 to 14 minutes
Beets, large, whole	20 minutes
Broccoli	2 to 3 minutes
Brussels sprouts	4 minutes
Cabbage, shredded or wedges	2 to 3 minutes
Carrots, sliced or small	4 to 5 minutes
Cauliflower, florets	2 to 3 minutes
Chestnuts (in shell, scored)	6 minutes
Corn, on the cob	3 minutes
Eggplant, cubed	2 to 3 minutes
Kale or other sturdy greens	2 minutes
Potatoes, sliced or cubed (use waxy red potatoes, unless for mashed)	5 to 6 minutes
Potatoes, whole, unpeeled, small to medium	5 to 15 minutes
Potatoes, sweet, cubed	5 minutes
Pumpkin or winter squash	5 to 7 minutes
Rutabagas or turnips, cubed	4 to 5 minutes
Zucchini, sliced	1 minute

FRUIT	*cooked with 1/2 cup (125 mL) water, wine or juice*
Apples, fresh	3 to 4 minutes
Apricots, fresh	2 minutes
Apricots, dried	4 minutes
Figs (dried)	6 minutes
Berries, cherries	0 minutes (bring to pressure and remove from heat)
Peaches, fresh, halved	2 to 3 minutes
Pears, fresh, halved	3 to 4 minutes
Prunes, dried	5 to 6 minutes

MEAT AND POULTRY	COOKING TIME (APPROX.)	COOKING LIQUID
Beef, stew meat, cubed	20 to 30 minutes	1 cup (250 mL)
Beef, roast or brisket, 3 lbs (1.5 kg)	35 to 45 minutes	1 to 2 cups (250 to 500 mL)
Beef/veal, shanks	45 minutes	1 cup (250 mL)
Corned beef	50 to 60 minutes	2 to 3 cups (500 to 750 mL)
Beef round steak, 1/2 inch (1 cm) thick	15 to 20 minutes	1 cup (250 mL)
Beef short ribs	25 minutes	1 1/2 to 2 cups (375 to 500 mL)
Ham, picnic shoulder, uncooked, 3 lbs (1.5 kg)	30 minutes	2 cups (500 mL)
Ham, slices, uncooked, 1 inch (2.5 cm) thick	12 minutes	1 cup (250 mL)
Pork chops, 1/2 inch (1 cm) thick	9 minutes	1 cup (250 mL)
Pork shoulder or butt roast, 3 lbs (1.5 kg)	40 to 50 minutes	1 1/2 cups (375 mL)
Pork spare ribs, 2 lbs (1 kg)	15 minutes	1 to 2 cups (250 to 500 mL)
Pork loin roast, 3 lbs (1.5 kg)	30 to 40 minutes	1 1/2 cups (375 mL)
Lamb, shoulder roast, 3 lbs (1.5 kg)	35 to 40 minutes	1 cup (250 mL)
Lamb, leg roast, 3 lbs (1.5 kg)	35 to 45 minutes	2 cups (500 mL)
Lamb, shoulder cubed	15 to 20 minutes	1 cup (250 mL)
Chicken, whole, 2 to 3 lbs (1 to 1.5 kg)	20 to 25 minutes	1 cup (250 mL)
Chicken pieces, 2 to 3 lbs (1 to 1.5 kg)	15 to 20 minutes	1 cup (250 mL)
Cornish hens, 2	10 to 12 minutes	1 cup (250 mL)
Duck, pieces	15 minutes	1 cup (250 mL)
Turkey, breast, whole, 5 to 6 lbs (2.5 to 3 kg)	35 to 45 minutes	3 cups (750 mL)
Turkey legs and thighs	45 to 55 minutes	3 cups (750 mL)

GRAINS	COOKING TIME (APPROX.) *plus time for natural pressure release*	WATER *use for jiggle-top models*
Amaranth	4 minutes	1 1/2 to 1 3/4* cups (375 to 450 mL)
Barley, hulled	35 to 40 minutes	3 cups (750 mL)
Barley, pearl or pot	16 to 20 minutes	3 cups (750 mL)
Buckwheat	4 minutes	1 3/4 cups (425 mL)
Kamut	40 to 45 minutes	3 cups (750 mL)
Millet	12 minutes	1 3/4 to 2* cups (425 to 500 mL)
Quinoa	1 minute	1 1/2 cups (375 mL)
Rice, brown	25 minutes	1 1/2 to 1 3/4* cups (375 to 425 mL)
Rice, wild	22 to 25 minutes	3 cups (750 mL)
Rice, white	5 to 6 minutes	1 1/2 to 1 3/4 cups
Risotto	6 to 7 minutes	2 1/4 cups (550 mL)
Rye berries	25 to 30 minutes	3 cups (750 mL)
Spelt	35 to 45 minutes	3 cups (750 mL)
Wheat berries	35 to 46 minutes	3 cups (750 mL)

BEANS soaked overnight or pressure-soaked (* unless otherwise indicated)	COOKING TIME (APPROX.) plus time for natural pressure release	WATER add 1 tbsp (15 mL) vegetable oil
Adzuki (Japanese brown)	5 to 6 minutes	3 cups (750 mL)
Anasazi	5 to 6 minutes	3 cups (750 mL)
Appaloosa	8 to 10 minutes	3 cups (750 mL)
Baby lima or butter bean	5 to 6 minutes	3 cups (750 mL)
Black	8 to 9 minutes	3 cups (750 mL)
Black-eyed peas, no soaking*	10 minutes	3 cups (750 mL)
Cannellini (white)	8 to 10 minutes	3 cups (750 mL)
Chickpea (garbanzo)	10 to 15 minutes	3 cups (750 mL)
Christmas lima	6 to 8 minutes	3 cups (750 mL)
Cranberry (barlotto)	6 to 8 minutes	3 cups (750 mL)
Fava	12 to 15 minutes	3 cups (750 mL)
Flageolet	8 to 10 minutes	3 cups (750 mL)
Great Northern	8 to 10 minutes	3 cups (750 mL)
Lentils, brown, no soaking*	10 minutes	Cover by 2 inches (5 cm)
Lentils, French, no soaking*	12 minutes	Cover by 2 inches (5 cm)
Lentils, red, no soaking*	5 minutes	Cover by 2 inches (5 cm)
Lima, large	4 to 6 minutes	3 cups (750 mL)
Navy	4 to 5 minutes	3 cups (750 mL)
Peas, split, no soaking*	8 to 10 minutes	3 cups (750 mL)
Peas, whole	5 to 8 minutes	3 cups (750 mL)
Pigeon peas	5 to 8 minutes	3 cups (750 mL)
Pinto	4 to 6 minutes	3 cups (750 mL)
Rattlesnake	4 to 6 minutes	3 cups (750 mL)
Scarlet runner	8 to 10 minutes	3 cups (750 mL)
Soybean, white	10 to 14 minutes	3 cups (750 mL)
Soybean, black	16 to 18 minutes	3 cups (750 mL)
Tongues of fire	8 to 10 minutes	3 cups (750 mL)

Acknowledgements

My first thank you is to all the people at Coranco for their co-operation, without which my recipe testers and I would not have been able to develop and refine these recipes. Everything in *The Best Pressure Cooker Recipes* was tested in the Lagostina Brava Plus and Logica models. They are both first-class pressure cookers, but my real favorite is the Logica, with its handy pressure release valve, easy-opening lid and dual pressure settings. This model is stylish, very versatile and dependable, and it will give you years of great performance in the kitchen.

I would also like to thank my main recipe tester, Susan Spicer, for her endless hours of hard work. Without her help, this project could not have been completed on time, and with such success.

These recipes were developed and tested in Calgary at an altitude of nearly 3,500 feet. They were then re-tested at an altitude of 650 feet. We believe that all of the recipes can be prepared with the cooking times as set out in any pressure cooker at any altitude. However, see pages 12 to 13 for a more detailed description of some of the adjustments you may want to make in certain conditions.

I hope these recipes give you both inspiration and years of enjoyment with pressure cooking.

Cinda Chavich

Appetizers

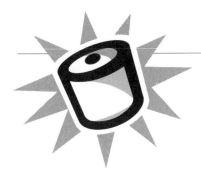

Hummus

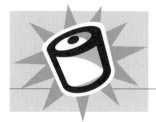

Makes 3 cups (750 mL)

This Mediterranean spread is perfect with warm triangles of pita bread or veggies for dipping.

This is a good, basic recipe for hummus. When you want a change in flavor and color, try adding 1/2 cup (125 mL) roasted red pepper or 1/2 cup (125 mL) chopped parsley (or even roasted garlic) before puréeing the mixture.

1 cup	dried chickpeas	250 mL
1 tsp	ground cumin	5 mL
1 tsp	salt	5 mL
1/4 cup	extra virgin olive oil	50 mL
1/4 cup	tahini paste (sesame seed paste)	50 mL
2 tsp	sesame oil	10 mL
	Juice of 2 large lemons	
3	cloves garlic, minced	3
1/4 cup	warm water (approximate)	50 mL

1. Soak chickpeas overnight in water to cover or use the quick pressure-soak method, page 130. Drain.

2. In a pressure cooker, cover chickpeas with at least 1 inch (2.5 cm) water. Lock the lid in place and bring cooker up to full pressure over high heat. Reduce heat to medium-low, just to maintain even pressure, and cook for 15 minutes. Remove from heat and release pressure quickly. Drain.

3. In a food processor, combine chickpeas, cumin, salt, olive oil, tahini, sesame oil, lemon juice and garlic; purée until smooth. If mixture seems too dry, add enough of the warm water as necessary to thin. Serve immediately with warm pita bread or refrigerate.

Dhal Dip with Pappadums

Makes about 2 cups (500 mL)

This is the perfect starter for an Indian meal. Serve the spicy split-pea spread with crispy pappadums and sliced peppers, green beans and zucchini sticks for dipping. Or spread it on a pita and top with grilled vegetables for an exotic vegetarian wrap.

TIP

To puff pappadums, fry them in hot oil for a few seconds or cook them in the microwave for about 45 seconds. You can buy large round pappadums or tiny cocktail-sized crackers.

1 tbsp	olive oil	15 mL
1 tsp	butter	5 mL
1	small onion, chopped	1
2 tsp	minced ginger root	10 mL
1	clove garlic, minced	1
1	serrano chili pepper, seeded and minced	1
1/2 tsp	garam masala	2 mL
1/4 tsp	ground turmeric	1 mL
1/2 tsp	dry mustard	2 mL
1 cup	dried yellow split peas	250 mL
2 cups	water	500 mL
1/4 cup	plain yogurt *or* sour cream	50 mL
2 tbsp	chopped cilantro	25 mL

1. In a pressure cooker, heat oil and butter over medium heat. Add onion, ginger, garlic and serrano chili; sauté until soft. Stir in garam masala, turmeric and dry mustard; cook for 1 minute or until spices are fragrant. Stir in split peas and add water.

2. Lock the lid in place and bring cooker up to full pressure over high heat. Reduce heat to medium-low, just to maintain even pressure, and cook for 8 minutes. Remove from the heat; allow pressure to drop naturally. Transfer to a bowl.

3. Stir *dhal* until cooled and thickened. Whisk in yogurt until mixture is smooth; stir in cilantro. Serve with pappadums for dipping.

Spiced Chickpeas

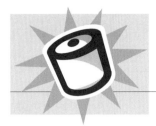

*Makes 2 to 3 cups
(500 to 750 mL)*

Here, cooked chickpeas are slowly sautéed with Indian spices until they are golden brown and crisp. This addictive vegetarian snack is great served with beer or cocktails.

1 cup	dried chickpeas	250 mL
4 cups	water	1 L
1	small onion, peeled	1
1	bay leaf	1
1/4 cup	butter	50 mL
2 tbsp	olive oil	25 mL
1 tsp	minced garlic	5 mL
1 tsp	onion salt	5 mL
1 tsp	ground ginger	5 mL
1 tsp	ground turmeric	5 mL
1/2 tsp	ground coriander	2 mL
1/4 tsp	cayenne pepper (or to taste)	1 mL
1 tbsp	kosher salt	15 mL

1. Soak chickpeas overnight in water to cover or use the quick pressure-soaking method, page 130. Drain.

2. In a pressure cooker, combine chickpeas, water, onion and bay leaf. Lock the lid in place and bring cooker up to full pressure over high heat. Reduce heat to medium-low, just to maintain even pressure, and cook for 15 minutes. Remove from heat; allow pressure to drop naturally. Drain chickpeas well; discard onion and bay leaf.

3. In a small pot over medium heat or in a bowl in the microwave, melt butter; stir in olive oil and garlic. In a large bowl, toss the chickpeas with the garlic mixture. Combine the onion salt, ginger, turmeric, coriander and cayenne; sprinkle spice mixture over chickpeas and toss to coat.

4. Spread chickpeas in a single layer on one or two large rimmed baking sheets. Bake in a preheated 400° F (200° C) oven for 5 to 10 minutes until brown and crisp, shaking the pan or stirring the peas often so that they brown evenly and don't burn. Transfer to a large bowl; toss with kosher salt.

5. Serve chickpeas hot or at room temperature. To reheat, spread on a rimmed baking sheet and bake in a preheated 350° F (180° C) oven for 5 to 10 minutes.

White Bean Dip

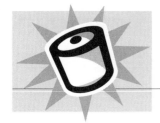

*Makes about 2 cups
(500 mL)*

With the addition of olive oil, garlic and chilies, the humble white bean becomes a zesty dip.

TIP

For a slightly more Mediterranean version, substitute dried thyme for cumin and chopped basil for cilantro. Gently heat the dip to warm it, then mix in a few ounces of crumbled goat cheese or feta cheese and serve with pita wedges.

3/4 cup	dried white beans, such as Great Northern or navy beans	175 mL
2	cloves garlic	2
3 tbsp	lemon juice	45 mL
1/3 cup	extra virgin olive oil	75 mL
2 tsp	ground cumin	10 mL
1 1/2 tsp	chili powder	7 mL
Pinch	red pepper flakes	Pinch
	Salt and freshly ground black pepper to taste	
3 tbsp	minced cilantro	45 mL

1. Soak beans overnight in water to cover or use the quick pressure-soaking method, page 130. Drain.

2. In a pressure cooker, cover beans with at least 1 inch (2.5 cm) water. Lock the lid in place and bring cooker up to full pressure over high heat. Reduce heat to medium-low, just to maintain even pressure, and cook for 12 to 13 minutes for Great Northern beans or 8 to 9 minutes for navy beans. Remove from heat and allow pressure to drop naturally. Drain beans and rinse under cold running water to cool them quickly.

3. In a food processor, drop cloves of garlic through feed tube with machine running to chop. Add beans, lemon juice, olive oil, cumin, chili powder and red pepper flakes; purée until smooth.

4. Fold in cilantro and season to taste with salt and pepper. Serve with taco chips or fresh vegetables.

Braised Artichokes with Red Pepper Aïoli

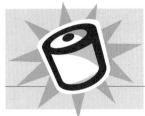

Serves 4 to 6

The flavors in this dish remind me of the south of France, where thyme and rosemary grow wild and perfume the air. It makes the perfect first course for a special Mediterranean meal.

The artichokes are eaten by pulling the leaves off, one by one, then drawing them through your teeth to remove the tender flesh at the base of each leaf. Be sure to supply a dish for leaf discards and finger bowls for this hands-on appetizer.

TIP

If you don't have time to roast peppers, use a prepared red pepper spread (such as Gloria brand).

RED PEPPER AÏOLI

1	clove garlic, minced	1
1/4 tsp	salt	1 mL
1/4 tsp	white pepper	1 mL
Pinch	cayenne pepper	Pinch
1	egg yolk	1
1/4 cup	roasted red bell pepper (see Tip, at left, for alternative)	50 mL
1 tbsp	lemon juice	15 mL
1/3 cup	extra virgin olive oil	75 mL
	Juice of 2 lemons	
4 cups	water	1 L
12	small artichokes	12
2 tbsp	olive oil	25 mL
6	shallots, peeled and halved	6
4	cloves garlic, minced	4
1	sprig rosemary, leaves minced	1
1/2 tsp	salt	2 mL
1/2 tsp	freshly ground black pepper	2 mL
1/2 tsp	dried thyme	2 mL
1/2 cup	diced fresh or canned tomatoes	125 mL
1/2 cup	chicken stock	125 mL
1/3 cup	red wine *or* tomato juice	75 mL
2 tbsp	balsamic vinegar	25 mL

1. RED PEPPER AÏOLI: In a food processor, combine garlic, salt, white pepper, cayenne, egg yolk, red pepper and lemon juice; purée until smooth. With machine running, slowly add oil through the feed tube, until the aïoli is thick and emulsified. Refrigerate until ready to serve.

2. In a large bowl, add juice of one of the lemons to water. Cut stems from artichokes, trim tips of leaves and cut each artichoke in half lengthwise. Scoop out choke and place artichoke halves in lemon water to prevent discoloration.

3. In a pressure cooker, heat oil over medium heat. Add shallots and garlic; sauté until they begin to color. Stir in rosemary, salt, pepper, thyme, tomatoes, stock, wine and vinegar. Drain artichokes and add to cooker. Pour remaining lemon juice over top.

4. Lock the lid in place and bring cooker up to full pressure over high heat. Reduce heat to medium-low, just to maintain even pressure, and cook for 7 minutes. Remove from heat; release pressure quickly.

5. With a slotted spoon, transfer artichokes to a deep serving dish. Boil braising liquid until it's reduced by half. Strain sauce over artichokes and let cool to room temperature. Serve artichokes as a side dish or on individual plates, drizzled generously with the red pepper aïoli.

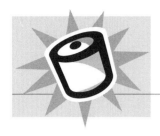

Sun-Dried Tomato Cheesecake

7- OR 8-INCH (1.5 OR 2 L) SPRINGFORM PAN (USE SMALLER SIZE IF NECESSARY TO FIT INSIDE PRESSURE COOKER)

RACK OR TRIVET TO FIT BOTTOM OF PRESSURE COOKER

Serves 8 to 10

Serve this savory "cheesecake" spread on thin slices of baguette. It makes a pretty addition to an appetizer buffet or cheese tray – cut it into pie-shaped wedges and serve with a cheese knife alongside your favorite ripe Brie.

Cheesecake can be wrapped and refrigerated for up to 3 days or frozen for up to 3 months.

TIP

Don't discard the oil from your sun-dried tomatoes. It's great for salad dressings or brushing over meat and fish before grilling.

CRUST

3 tbsp	butter, softened	45 mL
1/3 cup	breadcrumbs *or* crushed onion crackers	75 mL

FILLING

1/2 cup	sun-dried tomatoes in oil, drained, oil reserved	125 mL
6	cloves garlic, minced	6
2 tbsp	chopped oregano (or 1 tsp [5 mL] dried)	25 mL
3	eggs	3
3 tbsp	all-purpose flour	45 mL
12 oz	cream cheese, softened	375 g
4 oz	goat cheese, softened	125 g
1/4 cup	sour cream *or* plain yogurt	50 mL
1/2 cup	chopped green onions	125 mL
2 cups	water	500 mL

TOPPING

1/2 cup	sour cream	125 mL

Baguette or crackers for serving

1. CRUST: Thickly butter bottom and sides of springform pan. Sprinkle breadcrumbs inside pan, tilting to coat the sides. Leave excess crumbs on bottom. Wrap outside of pan with foil to seal. Set aside.

2. FILLING: In a food processor, purée sun-dried tomatoes with 1 tbsp (15 mL) of the reserved oil, garlic, oregano and eggs. Add flour, cream cheese, goat cheese and sour cream; purée until smooth. Stir in green onions. Pour mixture into prepared pan and cover with foil, making sure pan is well sealed.

3. Set rack in bottom of pressure cooker. Pour in water. Fold a 2-foot (60 cm) length of foil several times to make a strip that will be used to remove pan. Center pan on mid-point of strip and fold the ends together to make a handle. Use strip to lower pan into the cooker.

4. Lock lid in place and bring cooker up to full pressure over high heat. Reduce heat to medium-low, just to maintain even pressure, and cook for 20 minutes. Remove from heat; let pressure drop naturally for 7 minutes. Release remaining pressure with quick-release valve. Let cheesecake cool in cooker for a few minutes. Using foil handle, lift pan out of cooker onto cooling rack. Remove foil lid. Cheesecake should be set around edges, but still slightly loose in center. If center is still liquid, seal with foil and return to cooker. Lock lid in place. Bring up to full pressure over high heat. Reduce heat to medium-low, just to maintain even pressure, and cook for 2 minutes longer. When cheesecake is cooked, remove foil. Use a paper towel to mop up any water pooled on top of cake.

5. TOPPING: In a small bowl, whisk sour cream with another 1 tbsp (15 mL) of the reserved oil. Spread over cheesecake, smoothing top. Let cool to room temperature. Refrigerate for at least 8 hours or overnight before serving.

6. With a knife dipped in hot water, cut cheesecake into quarters and present with a cheese knife and sliced baguette.

Beef- and Rice-Stuffed Grape Leaves

Makes about 30
Serves 6 as a main
course

Sue Spicer, the devoted home economist who helped test most of the recipes for this book, thought that the pressure cooker would be perfect for making one of her favorite Greek appetizers, stuffed grape leaves (or *dolmades*). She was right. The pressure cooker cuts the cooking time down to 15 minutes (from 1 1/2 hours in the oven), and creates perfectly tender *dolmades*. This is her delicious recipe, which makes about 30 stuffed leaves. They can be served hot as a main course or at room temperature as an appetizer.

Try the pressure cooking method used here with your favorite recipe for cabbage rolls. It's a winner.

1 lb	lean ground beef	500 g
1 cup	long grain rice	250 mL
1	roasted red bell pepper, minced	1
1	onion, minced	1
1 cup	beef stock	250 mL
1/3 cup	olive oil	75 mL
2 tbsp	finely chopped mint	25 mL
1 tsp	dried tarragon	5 mL
1/2 tsp	salt	2 mL
1/2 tsp	freshly ground black pepper	2 mL
30	grape leaves (about 1 small jar)	30
2 cups	water	500 mL
2 tbsp	lemon juice	25 mL

SAUCE

2	eggs, beaten	2
1 tbsp	olive oil	15 mL
2 tbsp	lemon juice	25 mL
2 tsp	Dijon mustard	10 mL
1 tsp	granulated sugar	5 mL

1. In a large bowl, combine beef, rice, red pepper, onion, stock, oil, mint, tarragon, salt and pepper. Drain grape leaves; carefully separate and rinse in cold water. Pat leaves dry. Place any damaged leaves in the bottom of pressure cooker.

2. Arrange leaves, dull-side up, on work surface. Place 2 tbsp (25 mL) of filling on each leaf. Fold stem-end over filling, turn in the sides and loosely roll, allowing room for rice to expand while cooking.

3. Arrange stuffed leaves in the cooker in layers. Do not pack too tightly. Pour water and lemon juice over leaves.

4. Lock lid in place and bring cooker up to full pressure over high heat. Reduce heat to medium-low, just to maintain even pressure, and cook for 15 minutes. Remove from heat and allow pressure to drop naturally. Carefully transfer cooked *dolmades* to a serving platter.

5. SAUCE: In a heavy saucepan over low heat, whisk together eggs, oil, lemon juice, mustard; cook, stirring constantly, for about 5 to 10 minutes until thick. For appetizers, serve sauce in a bowl alongside the stuffed grape leaves for dipping. As a main course, add water as necessary to thin the sauce to pouring consistency and drizzle over *dolmades*.

Moroccan Chicken Meatballs with Creamy Tomato Sauce

Serves 4 to 6

These meatballs make a nice hot hors d'oeuvre on a party buffet table. Or serve the meatballs and creamy sauce over pasta or instant couscous for a simple family supper.

1	onion	1
1/4 cup	packed parsley leaves	50 mL
1/4 cup	packed cilantro leaves	50 mL
1/4 cup	packed mint leaves	50 mL
1 1/2 lbs	lean ground chicken	750 g
1	egg	1
1/2 tsp	ground cumin	2 mL
1/2 tsp	sweet paprika	2 mL
1/2 tsp	salt	2 mL
1/4 tsp	ground cinnamon	1 mL
1/4 to 1/2 tsp	cayenne pepper	1 to 2 mL

SAUCE

2 tbsp	olive oil	25 mL
1	onion, sliced	1
1	clove garlic, minced	1
2 tbsp	all-purpose flour	25 mL
1	can (28 oz [796 mL]) tomatoes, crushed or puréed	1
1	can (10 oz [284 mL]) chicken broth, undiluted	1
1 tsp	sweet paprika	5 mL
1/4 cup	whipping (35%) cream	50 mL
	Salt and freshly ground black pepper to taste	

1. In a food processor, combine onion, parsley, cilantro and mint; pulse until finely minced. In a bowl, using your hands, mix onion mixture, chicken, egg, cumin, paprika, cinnamon, salt and cayenne until well blended. Cover and refrigerate for 1 hour. Shape meat mixture into 25 small meatballs.

2. SAUCE: In a pressure cooker, heat oil over medium-low heat. Add onion and garlic; sauté for about 10 minutes or until onion is golden brown and caramelized. Add flour and cook, stirring, for 1 minute. Stir in tomatoes, chicken broth and paprika; bring to a boil. Carefully add meatballs to sauce.

3. Lock lid in place and bring cooker up to full pressure over high heat. Reduce heat to medium-low, just to maintain even pressure, and cook for 10 minutes. Remove from heat and release pressure quickly. Gently stir in cream and season to taste with salt and pepper.

Eggplant Caponata

Makes 4 cups (1 L)

Caponata is the Sicilian version of French ratatouille. Serve it on toasts for an hors d'oeuvre or tossed with hot pasta for a speedy main course.

TIP

Salting eggplant and rinsing away the brown juices that rise to the surface is necessary to eliminate bitterness. This step is not necessary if you use smaller Japanese eggplants.

1	large eggplant, skin on, cut into 1-inch (2.5 cm) cubes	1
2 tsp	salt	10 mL
1 tbsp	packed brown sugar	15 mL
2 tbsp	tomato paste	25 mL
2 tbsp	balsamic vinegar	25 mL
1/2 cup	olive oil	125 mL
1	onion, chopped	1
1	small red bell pepper, chopped	1
1	small yellow bell pepper, chopped	1
1 cup	canned crushed tomatoes	250 mL
1/2 cup	air-cured black olives, pitted and chopped	125 mL
2 tbsp	chopped basil	25 mL

1. Toss eggplant with salt; transfer to a colander and let stand for 30 minutes. Rinse and drain well. Pat dry with paper towels.

2. In a bowl whisk together sugar, tomato paste and vinegar; set aside.

3. In a pressure cooker, heat oil over high heat. Add eggplant and sauté for 2 minutes. Stir in onion, red and yellow peppers and tomatoes. Lock lid in place and bring cooker up to full pressure over high heat. Reduce heat to medium-low, just to maintain even pressure, and cook for 4 to 5 minutes. Remove from heat and release pressure quickly.

4. Stir to break up eggplant slightly. Stir in reserved tomato-paste mixture, olives and basil. Allow to cool. Serve at room temperature or chilled. (It will keep, covered, in the refrigerator for up to 4 days.)

DHAL DIP WITH PAPPADUMS (PAGE 21) ➤

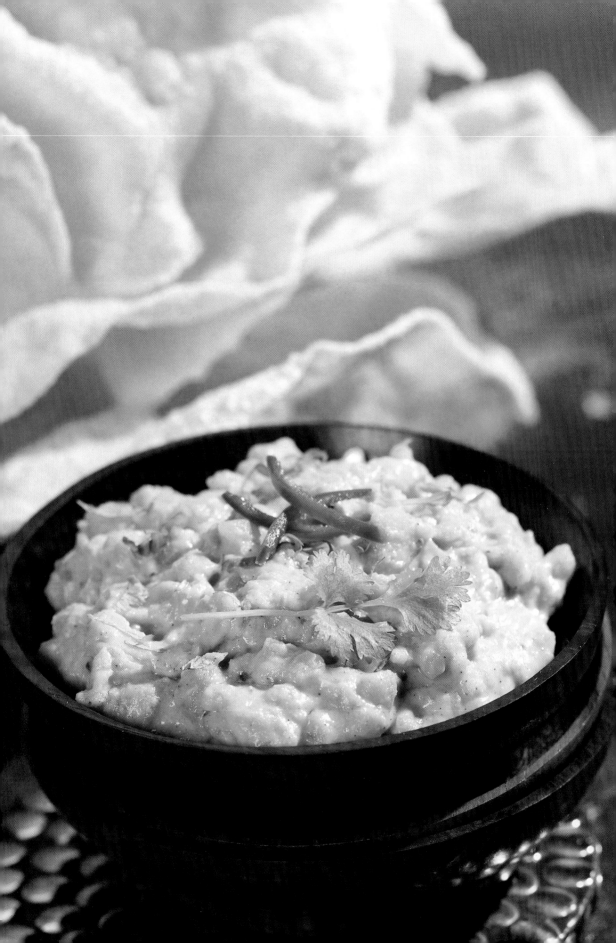

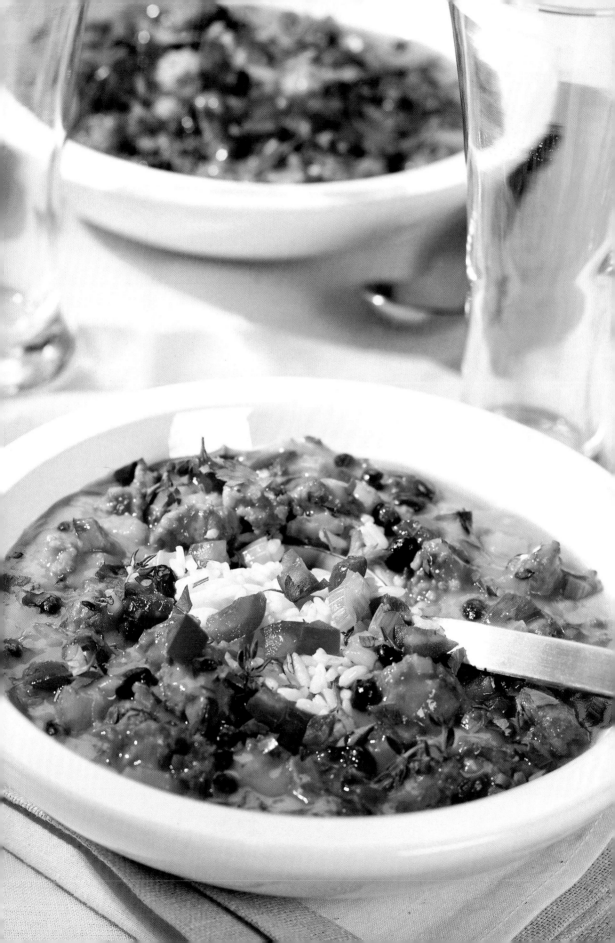

Soups

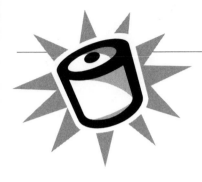

Spicy Sweet Potato Soup

Serves 4

This soup is creamy, rich and smooth – but has hardly any added fat. The gorgeous orange color makes it the perfect prelude to a fall supper.

Garam masala is a spice mixture that's available at Indian groceries and in the spice sections of larger supermarkets. If it's not available, substitute your favorite curry powder.

1 tbsp	olive oil	15 mL
2	cloves garlic, minced	2
1	onion, chopped	1
3 cups	chicken stock	750 mL
2 cups	chopped peeled sweet potatoes	500 mL
1	small potato, peeled and chopped	1
2	carrots, chopped	2
1	ancho chili, stem and seeds removed	1
1 1/2 tsp	garam masala	7 mL
	Salt to taste	

1. In a pressure cooker, heat oil over medium heat. Add garlic and onion; sauté for 5 minutes or until soft. Stir in stock, sweet potatoes, potato, carrots, and ancho chili.

2. Lock the lid in place and bring cooker up to full pressure over high heat. Reduce heat to medium-low, just to maintain even pressure, and cook for 12 minutes. Remove from heat and release pressure quickly.

3. Purée soup with an immersion blender or in a food processor until creamy and smooth. Stir in garam masala and season with salt to taste.

Mexican Pinto Bean Soup

Serves 4 to 6

Hearty and filling, this soup is the perfect anti-dote to a case of the mid-winter blues.

1 cup	dried pinto beans	250 mL
2	cloves garlic	2
1	large onion, halved	1
1 tbsp	vegetable oil	15 mL
1 tsp	salt	5 mL
2 tbsp	olive oil *or* vegetable oil	25 mL
1/3 cup	whipping (35%) cream	75 mL
	Grated Monterey Jack cheese, cilantro sprigs and diced avocado for garnish	

1. Soak beans overnight in water to cover or use quick pressure-soak method, page 130. Drain.

2. In a pressure cooker, cover beans with at least 1 inch (2.5 cm) water. Add 1 clove garlic, half the onion and the vegetable oil. Lock the lid in place and bring cooker up to full pressure over high heat. Reduce heat to medium-low, just to maintain even pressure, and cook for 10 minutes. Remove from heat and release pressure quickly. The beans should be very soft. If not, lock the lid in place and return to full pressure; cook for 2 to 3 minutes longer. Remove from heat and release pressure quickly. Drain beans, reserving cooking liquid.

3. In a food processor, purée bean mixture, adding some of the reserved liquid as necessary to make smooth.

4. Meanwhile, mince remaining onion and garlic. In a large pot, heat oil over medium heat. Add onion and garlic; sauté for about 5 minutes or until golden. Add puréed bean mixture to the pot along with enough of the reserved liquid to make a smooth soup.

5. Bring to a boil and simmer for 10 minutes. Season with salt and pepper. Add cream and simmer until thickened and smooth. Serve individual bowls of soup topped with a handful of grated cheese, a few cubes of avocado and a sprig of cilantro.

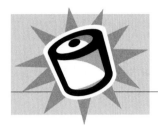

Root Vegetable Soup

Serves 4

Flavorful root vegetables are available at all times of the year for this creamy, elegant soup, which is deceptively low in fat. If you're using dried dill, add it before pressure cooking.

TIP

For a spicy garnish to this (or any other) creamy soup, place 3 dried ancho chilies in a bowl and add boiling water to cover; soak for 30 minutes. Drain, remove stems and seeds, and purée chilies with 1/4 cup (50 mL) chicken stock until smooth. Combine with enough low-fat sour cream to make a smooth sauce. Pour the sauce into a squeeze bottle and use to garnish soups with decorative swirls or simply drizzle it from a spoon. Use the ancho cream to finish this soup, bean soup, pumpkin soup or other creamy concoctions for a blast of chili flavor.

2 tsp	vegetable oil *or* butter	10 mL
1	clove garlic, minced	1
1 cup	chopped onions	250 mL
3 cups	chicken stock	750 mL
1	potato, peeled and chopped	1
3/4 cup	chopped carrots	175 mL
3/4 cup	peeled chopped sweet potato	175 mL
1/2 cup	chopped parsnip	125 mL
2 tbsp	chopped dill (or 2 tsp [10 mL] dried)	25 mL

Salt and white pepper to taste

1. In a pressure cooker, heat oil over medium heat. Add garlic and onion; sauté for about 5 minutes or until tender. Add stock, potato, carrot, sweet potato and parsnip.

2. Lock the lid in place and bring cooker up to full pressure over high heat. Reduce heat to medium-low, just to maintain even pressure, and cook for 7 minutes. Remove from heat and release pressure quickly.

3. In a food processor or with an immersion blender, purée vegetables with some of the cooking liquid until smooth. Return purée to the pot and stir to mix with the remaining liquid. Bring to a boil. Stir in dill and season with salt and white pepper just before serving.

Scotch Broth

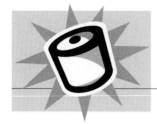

Serves 8

This is a classic Scottish dish, one of those old-fashioned, hearty soups that are perfect for serving on a winter day.

TIP

Next time you bone a leg of lamb, save the bones and brown them. Use in this recipe along with the meat to give the soup a rich color and flavor. Remove bones from soup before serving.

2 tsp	vegetable oil	10 mL
3	stalks celery, diced	3
1	onion, diced	1
1 lb	boneless lamb shoulder or shank, trimmed of fat and finely chopped	500 g
8 cups	chicken stock *or* cold water	2 L
2 cups	carrots, cut in small dice	500 mL
2 cups	turnips, cut in small dice	500 mL
1 tsp	freshly ground black pepper	5 mL
1/2 tsp	dried thyme leaves	2 mL
2 tsp	minced garlic	10 mL
1	bay leaf	1
1 cup	pearl barley	250 mL
	Salt to taste	

1. In a pressure cooker, heat oil over medium heat. Add celery and onions; sauté for about 8 minutes or until soft. Add lamb, in batches, and brown on all sides. Return lamb and accumulated juices to cooker. Stir in stock, carrots, turnips, pepper, thyme, garlic and bay leaf. Stir in barley.

2. Lock the lid in place and bring cooker up to full pressure over high heat. Reduce heat to medium-low, just to maintain even pressure, and cook for 22 minutes. Remove from heat and allow pressure to drop naturally.

3. Season to taste with salt. Discard bay leaf before serving.

Thai Green Curry and Sweet Potato Soup

Serves 4

For an even spicier version of this flavorful Asian soup, use a Thai red curry paste instead of the green variety. Both are available in jars or packets at Asian markets or the Asian-food section of many large supermarkets.

To make this soup into a substantial meal, ladle it over cooked egg or rice noodles.

2 tbsp	vegetable oil	25 mL
3	red, yellow or orange bell peppers, cut into slivers	3
2	cloves garlic, minced	2
1	large onion, slivered	1
1 tbsp	Thai green curry paste	15 mL
2	sweet potatoes, peeled and cubed	2
1	can (14 oz [398 mL]) unsweetened coconut milk	1
1/4 cup	water	50 mL
1 tsp	lemon or lime juice	5 mL
1 cup	snow peas or green beans, cut into 1-inch lengths	250 mL
1 tbsp	chopped cilantro	15 mL

1. In a pressure cooker, heat oil over medium heat. Add peppers, garlic and onion; sauté for 5 minutes. Stir in curry paste and cook for 1 minute. Add sweet potatoes, coconut milk, water and lemon juice.

2. Lock the lid in place and bring cooker up to full pressure over medium-high heat. Reduce heat to medium-low, just to maintain even pressure, and cook for 3 minutes. Remove from heat and release pressure quickly.

3. Stir in snow peas, cover and cook (not under pressure) for 2 to 3 minutes or just until vegetables are tender-crisp. Stir in cilantro before serving.

Ham and Split Pea Soup

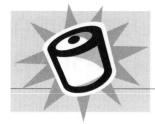

Serves 8

Split peas and red lentils reduce to a purée when cooked. This can clog the pressure valve of a jiggle-top pressure cooker, so be careful! If you own this type of cooker and hear loud hissing noises during cooking, remove it from the heat and quickly release pressure by running cold water over the lid. Check for any food clogging the vent, wash the lid thoroughly, then return it to the pot and continue cooking. Always allow the pressure to come down naturally when cooking these legumes to avoid clogging the pressure valve. In newer models of cookers, there are several backup safety systems to automatically release pressure if there is a clog in the primary valve system, so cooking these kinds of foods is no longer a problem.

1 tbsp	butter *or* vegetable oil	15 mL
2	cloves garlic, minced	2
1	onion, chopped	1
1 lb	dried split peas (about 2 cups [500 mL])	500 g
2	carrots, diced	2
1/2 tsp	dried thyme	2 mL
8 oz	smoked ham or lean back bacon, finely diced	250 g
6 cups	chicken stock	1.5 L
4 cups	water	1 L
2 cups	dry white wine	500 mL
1/2 cup	brown rice	125 mL
1	pkg (10 oz [300 g]) frozen green peas, thawed *or* equal amount of fresh garden peas, in season, cooked	1

Salt and freshly ground black pepper

1. In a pressure cooker, melt butter over medium heat. Add garlic and onion; sauté for about 5 minutes or until tender. Stir in split peas, carrots, thyme, ham, stock, water, wine and brown rice.

2. Lock the lid in place and bring cooker up to full pressure over high heat. Reduce heat to medium-low, just to maintain even pressure, and cook for 10 minutes. Remove from heat and allow pressure to drop naturally for 10 minutes, then release any remaining pressure.

3. Stir in green peas and season to taste with salt and pepper. Bring soup to a boil and serve immediately. Or chill overnight and reheat the next day – the soup will be even more flavorful.

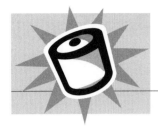

Red Bean and Ukrainian Sausage Soup

Serves 8

Brought to North America by Ukrainian immigrants over a century ago, smoky garlic ham sausage is a prairie staple.

TIP

If you can't find a good, garlicky ham sausage, substitute kielbasa in this hearty soup. For an even spicier version, choose chorizo.

1 1/2 cups	dried red kidney beans	375 mL
2	jalapeño peppers, chopped	2
1	large onion, chopped	1
8 oz	smoked Ukrainian ham sausage, chopped (see Tip, at left, for alternative)	250 g
1	bay leaf	1
1 tbsp	chili powder	15 mL
1 tsp	dried oregano	5 mL
1/2 tsp	freshly ground black pepper	2 mL
1/4 tsp	cayenne pepper	1 mL
3 cups	beef stock	750 mL
1	can (14 oz [398 mL]) plum tomatoes, crushed	1
1/2 cup	tomato sauce	125 mL
2 tbsp	packed brown sugar	25 mL

1. Soak beans in water to cover overnight or use the quick pressure-soak method, page 130. Drain.

2. In a pressure cooker, add water to cover beans by at least 1 inch (2.5 cm). Lock the lid in place and bring cooker up to full pressure over high heat. Reduce heat to medium-low, just to maintain even pressure, and cook for 12 minutes. Remove from heat and allow pressure to drop naturally. Drain beans and set aside.

3. Wipe pressure cooker clean and place over medium-high heat. Add jalapeño peppers, onion, sausage, bay leaf, chili powder, oregano, pepper and cayenne; cook, stirring, for 8 minutes or until the onions are soft. Stir in stock, tomatoes, tomato sauce, sugar and drained beans.

4. Lock the lid in place and bring cooker up to full pressure over high heat. Reduce heat to medium-low, just to maintain even pressure, and cook for 20 minutes. Remove from heat and allow pressure to drop naturally. Discard bay leaf before serving.

Beet and Vegetable Borscht

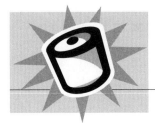

Serves 8

This is an old-fashioned soup, brought to Canada by immigrants from the Ukraine, Romania and other parts of Eastern Europe. For a vegetarian version, replace beef stock with water.

1 tbsp	butter	15 mL
2	cloves garlic, minced	2
1	large onion, minced	1
3 cups	cubed peeled potatoes (preferably a waxy red variety)	750 mL
1 cup	chopped carrots	250 mL
3 or 4	medium beets, unpeeled with 1 inch (2.5 cm) of tops intact	3 or 4
4 cups	shredded purple cabbage	1 L
8 cups	beef stock *or* water	2 L
1	can (14 oz [398 mL]) tomatoes, crushed	1
1 tbsp	balsamic or red wine vinegar	15 mL
	Salt to taste	
	Freshly ground black pepper to taste	
	Paprika to taste	
2 tbsp	chopped dill	25 mL
1/2 cup	sour cream	125 mL
2 tbsp	all-purpose flour	25 mL

1. In a pressure cooker, melt butter over medium heat. Add garlic and onion; sauté for about 5 minutes or until onion starts to brown. Stir in potatoes and carrots; sauté for 3 minutes. Add beets, cabbage, stock and tomatoes.

2. Lock the lid in place and bring cooker up to full pressure over high heat. Reduce heat to medium-low, just to maintain even pressure, and cook for 10 minutes. Remove from heat and allow pressure to drop naturally.

3. Transfer beets to a bowl and let cool slightly. Slip off skins, discard tops, and cut into cubes. Return beets to the soup and stir in the balsamic vinegar. Simmer for 10 minutes. Season to taste with salt, pepper and paprika. Stir in dill.

4. In a small bowl, whisk together sour cream and flour; stir into hot soup. Cook, stirring, for about 5 minutes or until hot (but not boiling) and slightly thickened. Serve immediately.

Pumpkin Soup

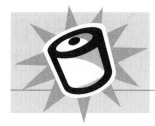

Serves 8

Start your next Thanksgiving meal with this classic seasonal soup. Use evaporated milk instead of cream to help to keep the fat content low, but without compromising the creamy texture or taste.

TIP

If you don't have fresh pumpkin, use 2 cups (500 mL) canned pumpkin purée (not pumpkin pie filling) and add it when you purée the soup in the food processor.

For an elegant garnish, artfully drizzle a little Ancho Chili Purée (see sidebar to recipe, page 36) over each serving using a plastic squeeze bottle.

1/4 cup	butter	50 mL
2	large onions, chopped	2
1	stalk celery, chopped	1
2	leeks, white parts only, chopped	2
3	large carrots, chopped	3
3	large potatoes, chopped	3
6 cups	chicken stock	1.5 L
2 cups	cubed peeled fresh pumpkin *or* canned pumpkin purée (see Tip, at left)	500 mL
1 1/2 cups	whipping (35%) cream *or* evaporated milk	375 mL
	Salt and freshly ground black pepper to taste	
2 tbsp	butter	25 mL
1/4 cup	chopped green onion	50 mL
1/4 cup	chopped parsley	50 mL

1. In a pressure cooker, melt 1/4 cup (50 mL) butter over medium heat. Add onions and celery; sauté for 5 minutes. Add leeks, carrots and potato; cook, stirring, for another 5 minutes. Stir in stock and pumpkin.

2. Lock the lid in place and bring cooker up to full pressure over high heat. Reduce heat to medium-low, just to maintain even pressure, and cook for 8 minutes. Remove from heat and release pressure quickly. Let cool slightly.

3. In a food processor, purée solids with some of the cooking liquid until smooth. Return purée to cooker and stir in cream. Heat through but don't boil. Season to taste with salt and pepper; whisk in butter until melted. Stir in green onions and parsley. Serve immediately.

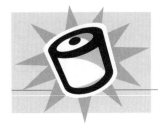

Moroccan Harira Soup with Chickpeas

Serves 4

The chili pepper gives this tomato-based soup a little zing. Choose a scotch bonnet pepper for a spicier version.

1/2 cup	dried chickpeas	125 mL
2 tbsp	olive oil	25 mL
1	large onion, chopped	1
1	chopped jalapeño or scotch bonnet pepper (the latter is hotter)	1
1/2 cup	chopped celery	125 mL
1 tsp	ground ginger	5 mL
1 tsp	ground turmeric	5 mL
1/2 tsp	ground cinnamon	2 mL
1/2 tsp	crumbled saffron (optional)	2 mL
1/2 tsp	freshly ground black pepper	2 mL
4 cups	water	1 L
3 cups	chopped tomatoes *or* 1 can (28 oz [796 mL]) crushed tomatoes	750 mL
1	can (10 oz [284 mL]) beef broth, undiluted	1
3/4 cup	green or brown lentils	175 mL
3 tbsp	lemon juice	45 mL
	Lemon slices for garnish	

1. Soak chickpeas overnight in water to cover or use the quick pressure-soak method, page 130. Drain.
2. In a pressure cooker, heat oil over medium heat. Add onion, jalapeño and celery; sauté for about 5 minutes or until soft. Stir in ginger, turmeric, cinnamon, saffron and pepper; cook for 1 minute until fragrant. Stir in chickpeas, water, tomatoes, broth, lentils and lemon juice, making sure cooker is no more than half full.
3. Lock the lid in place and bring cooker up to full pressure over high heat. Reduce heat to medium-low, just to maintain even pressure, and cook for 20 minutes. Remove from heat and allow pressure to drop naturally. Serve garnished with lemon slices.

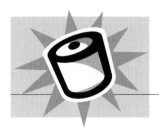

Cajun Black Bean and Sausage Gumbo

Serves 4 to 6

This hearty soup has an almost stew-like consistency. Serve it as a main course with cornbread and beer or ladle it over hot cooked rice in deep soup plates.

2 cups	dried black turtle beans	500 mL
7 cups	water	1.75 L
1/2 cup	vegetable oil	125 mL
1/2 cup	all-purpose flour	125 mL
2 lbs	spicy Italian sausage, casings removed, meat crumbled	1 kg
6	cloves garlic, minced	6
4	onions, chopped	4
4	stalks celery, chopped	4
1	red bell pepper, chopped	1
2 tsp	dried thyme	10 mL
4 cups	chicken stock	1 L
3 tbsp	Worcestershire sauce	45 mL
1/2 cup	minced parsley	125 mL
1/2 cup	chopped green onions	125 mL
	Salt and freshly ground black pepper to taste	
3 cups	cooked white rice	750 mL
1/2 cup	seeded chopped tomato	125 mL

1. Soak beans overnight in water to cover or use the quick pressure-soak method, page 130. Drain.

2. In a pressure cooker, combine beans and water. Lock the lid in place and bring cooker up to full pressure over high heat. Reduce heat to medium-low, just to maintain even pressure, and cook for 10 minutes. Remove from heat and allow pressure to drop naturally. Drain beans and set aside.

3. Wipe cooker clean and heat oil over medium-low heat; sprinkle in flour and cook, stirring constantly, until the *roux* turns the color of peanut butter, about 12 minutes. (Be careful – this gets very hot and burns easily.) Reduce heat to low. Stir in sausage, garlic, onions, celery, red pepper and thyme; cook, stirring, for about 10 minutes or until vegetables are very tender. Stir in beans, stock and Worcestershire.

4. Lock the lid in place and bring cooker up to full pressure over high heat. Reduce heat to medium-low, just to maintain even pressure, and cook for 8 minutes. Remove from heat and allow pressure to drop naturally. Stir in green onions and parsley; season to taste with salt and pepper.

5. Using a large spoon or ice cream scoop, place a big mound of rice in the center of each soup plate. Ladle soup around the rice. Garnish with chopped tomato.

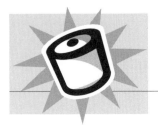

Spicy Mixed Bean and Barley Soup

Serves 6

This chunky vegetarian soup is perfect when you have a lot of different peas, beans and lentils to use up. Use the legumes called for in the recipe, or substitute whatever beans you have on hand.

For a hearty lunch, serve this soup with a biscuit or slice of homemade bread.

1 cup	mixed dried beans (red, white, black, pinto, black-eyed peas)	250 mL
1/2 cup	pearl or pot barley	125 mL
1/4 cup	green or yellow split peas	50 mL
1/4 cup	small red lentils	50 mL
2 tsp	ground cumin	10 mL
2 tsp	dried oregano	10 mL
1	bay leaf	1
1	small dried chili pepper, crumbled, *or* 1/2 tsp (2 mL) red pepper flakes	1
1 tsp	chili powder	5 mL
5 cups	cold water	1.25 L
2	cloves garlic, minced	2
1	stalk celery, chopped	1
1	onion, minced	1
1	can (14 oz [398 mL]) tomatoes, chopped	1
	Salt and freshly ground black pepper to taste	
2 tbsp	chopped parsley	25 mL

1. Soak beans overnight in water to cover or use the quick pressure-soak method, page 130. Drain.

2. In a pressure cooker, combine beans, barley, split peas, lentils, cumin, oregano, bay leaf, chili pepper, chili powder, water, garlic, celery, onion and tomatoes. Lock the lid in place and bring cooker up to full pressure over high heat. Reduce heat to medium-low, just to maintain even pressure, and cook for 20 minutes. Remove from heat and allow pressure to drop naturally. The beans and barley should be very tender. If not, lock the lid in place and bring to full pressure; cook for 5 minutes longer. Allow pressure to drop naturally.

3. Discard bay leaf. Season to taste with salt and pepper; stir in parsley.

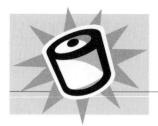

Wild Mushroom and Potato Bisque

Serves 4

There's very little cream in this elegant mushroom soup; it gets its smooth texture from potatoes. Make it without chicken stock for a vegetarian version. To speed things up even more, use the food processor to mince the vegetables and mushrooms.

TIP

If you have the time to prepare homemade stock, try the one used in BASIC RISOTTO (see recipe, page 142).

1 tbsp	olive oil	15 mL
2	cloves garlic, minced	2
1	small onion, minced	1
1	small tomato, seeded and chopped	1
1 cup	finely chopped wild and domestic mushrooms (brown, oyster, shiitake, Portobello, morels, cepes, etc.)	250 mL
12 oz	Yukon Gold potatoes (or other yellow-fleshed variety) peeled and grated	375 g
4 cups	chicken stock *or* vegetable stock (see Tip, at left)	1 L
1	bay leaf	1
3/4 tsp	minced thyme	4 mL
1/2 cup	whipping (35%) cream	125 mL
	Salt and freshly ground black pepper	

1. In a pressure cooker, heat oil over medium heat. Add garlic and onion; sauté for about 5 minutes or until soft. Add potato, tomato and mushrooms; cook, stirring, for about 5 minutes longer or until mushrooms begin to give up their moisture. Stir in the stock, bay leaf and thyme.

2. Lock the lid in place and bring cooker up to full pressure over high heat. Reduce heat to medium-low, just to maintain even pressure, and cook for 5 minutes. Release pressure quickly.

3. Discard bay leaf. Stir in cream and heat through. Using a potato masher, break up potatoes to thicken the soup, if necessary, or use an immersion blender to purée if you prefer a smoother soup. Season to taste with salt and pepper.

Pasta Fazool

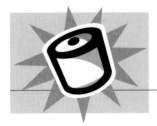

Serves 6

Is it a soup you eat with a fork – or a pasta dish to eat with a spoon? Either way, pasta fazool (or, strictly speaking, fagioli) makes a delicious one-pot meal. Add a loaf of bread, a jug of wine, and an après ski crowd.

1 1/2 cups	dried white cannellini beans	375 mL
3 tbsp	extra virgin olive oil	45 mL
2	stalks celery, chopped	2
1	large onion, chopped	1
1	carrot, chopped	1
4 oz	pancetta or prosciutto, finely chopped	125 g
1 tbsp	chopped garlic	15 mL
1 tbsp	chopped rosemary	15 mL
1 tsp	dried basil	5 mL
1/4 tsp	red pepper flakes	1 mL
1	can (14 oz [398 mL]) plum tomatoes, chopped	1
3 cups	chicken stock	750 mL
1 1/2 cups	dried short pasta (such as penne, small rotini or orecchiette)	375 mL
	Salt and freshly ground black pepper to taste	
	Extra virgin olive oil, rosemary sprigs and shards of Parmesan cheese for garnish	

1. Soak beans overnight in water to cover or use the quick pressure-soak method, page 130. Drain.

2. In a pressure cooker, heat oil over medium heat. Add celery, onion, carrot, pancetta and garlic; sauté until onion starts to brown. Stir in beans, rosemary, basil, red pepper flakes, tomatoes and stock.

3. Lock the lid in place and bring cooker up to full pressure over high heat. Reduce heat to medium-low, just to maintain even pressure, and cook for 15 minutes. Remove from heat and allow pressure to drop naturally. The beans should be very soft and starting to break down. If not, return to full pressure and cook for 1 to 2 minutes longer. Remove from heat and allow pressure to drop naturally.

4. Stir in pasta and simmer, uncovered, for 5 to 7 minutes or until pasta is tender. Serve in deep soup bowls. Garnish individual servings with a drizzle of olive oil, a sprig of rosemary and a few shards of Parmesan cheese.

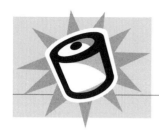

Winter Mushroom and Barley Soup

Serves 6

There's nothing delicate about this vegetarian soup – the portobello mushrooms and barley provide plenty of hearty flavor. For a richer (but non-vegetarian) soup, use beef or chicken broth instead of water.

2 tbsp	butter	25 mL
1 tbsp	olive oil	15 mL
1	large onion, halved and sliced	1
2	stalks celery, chopped	2
1	carrot, chopped	1
2 tsp	minced garlic	10 mL
1	bay leaf	1
1	portobello mushroom cap, chopped	1
8 oz	mixed fresh mushrooms, sliced	250 g
1/2 cup	pearl or pot barley	125 mL
6 cups	water	1.5 L
2 tbsp	vermouth *or* brandy	25 mL
2 tsp	salt	10 mL
1/4 tsp	freshly ground black pepper	1 mL
	Chopped parsley to garnish	

1. In a pressure cooker, heat butter and oil over medium heat. Add onion and sauté for 5 minutes or until softened. Stir in celery, carrot, garlic and bay leaf; cook, stirring, for 10 minutes or until onion begins to turn golden.

2. Add portobello and mixed mushrooms; cook for 5 minutes, until they release their moisture. Stir in the barley, water, vermouth, salt and pepper.

3. Lock the lid in place and bring cooker up to full pressure over high heat. Reduce heat to medium-low, just to maintain even pressure, and cook for 20 minutes. Remove from heat and allow pressure to drop naturally.

4. Discard bay leaf and adjust seasoning with salt and pepper to taste. Serve immediately, sprinkled with parsley.

Poultry

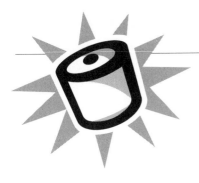

Chicken Stew with New Potatoes and Baby Carrots

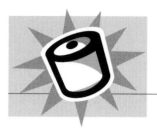

Serves 4 to 6

The dark meat of boneless chicken thighs is perfect in the pressure cooker and makes a classic, homestyle stew.

3 lbs	boneless skinless chicken thighs, cut into 2-inch (5 cm) chunks	1.5 kg
1 tbsp	vegetable oil	15 mL
1	large onion, minced	1
2	cloves garlic, minced	2
1 tbsp	all-purpose flour	15 mL
8 to 10	red new potatoes, halved (or quartered, if large)	8 to 10
3	stalks celery, diced	3
1	parsnip, peeled and diced	1
1	small turnip, peeled and diced	1
2 cups	baby carrots	500 mL
1 cup	chicken stock	250 mL
1/2 cup	dry white wine *or* sherry	125 mL
1	bay leaf	1
2 tbsp	chopped parsley	25 mL
1 tsp	chopped thyme (or 1/2 tsp [2 mL] dried)	5 mL
1 tsp	chopped sage (or 1/2 tsp [2 mL] dried)	5 mL
	Salt and freshly ground black pepper	

1. In a pressure cooker, heat oil over medium heat. Add chicken, in batches, and cook until browned. Set aside.

2. Drain off all but 1 tbsp (15 mL) of fat. Add onion and garlic; sauté for 2 minutes. Stir in flour, potatoes, celery, carrots, parsnip and turnip. Gradually stir in stock and wine. Add bay leaf. Bring to a boil and return chicken and any accumulated juices to cooker.

3. Lock the lid in place and bring cooker up to full pressure over high heat. Reduce heat to medium-low, just to maintain even pressure, and cook for 12 minutes. Remove from heat and release pressure quickly.

4. Discard bay leaf. Stir in parsley, thyme and sage. Season to taste with salt and pepper.

Chicken and Asian Noodles with Coconut Curry Sauce

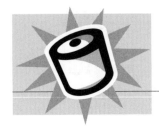

Serves 6

When you buy fresh cilantro, look for herbs with the roots attached; you can use them to infuse extra layers of flavor into this creamy curry sauce.

Thai green curry paste is sold in jars or foil pouches in Asian markets.

6	strips lemon zest	6
3	cilantro roots or stems	3
2	green Serrano chilies, halved lengthwise	2
2 lbs	boneless skinless chicken breasts or thighs, cut into strips	1 kg
2 to 3 tbsp	Thai green curry paste	25 to 45 mL
2 cups	light coconut milk	500 mL
1	small Asian eggplant, cut into small cubes	1
1 tbsp	packed brown sugar	15 mL
1/2 tsp	white pepper	2 mL
1/2 tsp	salt	2 mL
1 tbsp	fish sauce *(nam pla)*	15 mL
1 tsp	dark soy sauce	5 mL
1 tsp	lemon juice	5 mL
3	green onions, cut into thin strips	3
1/4 cup	chopped cilantro	50 mL
8 oz	fresh Chinese-style steamed egg noodles, cooked until tender and drained	250 g

1. Using kitchen string, tie lemon zest, cilantro roots or stems, and chilies into a bundle. Set aside.

2. In a pressure cooker over medium heat, sauté chicken and curry paste for 3 to 5 minutes or until chicken begins to brown. Stir in coconut milk, eggplant, brown sugar, pepper, salt, fish sauce, soy sauce, lemon juice and lemon-zest bundle.

3. Lock the lid in place and bring cooker up to full pressure over high heat. Reduce heat to medium-low, just to maintain even pressure, and cook for 8 minutes. Remove from heat and release pressure quickly.

4. Discard lemon-zest bundle. Simmer curry, uncovered, to thicken if necessary. Serve over noodles in deep bowls, sprinkled with green onions and cilantro.

Grandma's Sunday Chicken

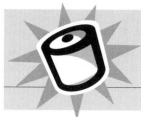

Serves 6

My grandmother used to treat us to her own version of chicken *pot-au-feu* every Sunday after church. Coming into her little house, you were enveloped in the steamy aroma of homemade chicken soup. She served her Sunday lunch in two stages – first, a rich chicken broth filled with hand-cut noodles; then the tender stewed chicken, carrots, parsnips and potatoes, drizzled with creamy dill sauce. My grandma got up very early on Sundays to make this magic – you can make it in the pressure cooker in 20 minutes.

8 to 10	small red potatoes, halved	8 to 10
4	large carrots, cut into large pieces	4
4	stalks celery, cut into large pieces	4
3	whole cloves garlic, peeled	3
2	onions, each cut into 6 pieces	2
2	parsnips, cut into large pieces	2
1	bay leaf	1
1 tbsp	chopped thyme (or 1 tsp [5 mL] dried)	15 mL
1 tsp	salt	5 mL
1 tsp	whole peppercorns	5 mL
1	3- to 4-lb (1.5 to 2 kg) chicken or stewing hen	1
6 cups	water *or* chicken stock	1.5 L
1 1/2 cups	small egg noodles	375 mL

DILL CREAM SAUCE

2 tbsp	butter	25 mL
2 tbsp	all-purpose flour	25 mL
3/4 cup	cream *or* milk	175 mL
2 tbsp	minced fresh dill (or 1 tsp [5 mL] dried)	25 mL
Pinch	paprika	Pinch
	Salt and freshly ground black pepper to taste	

1. In a pressure cooker, combine potatoes, carrots, celery, garlic, onions, parsnips, bay leaf, thyme, salt and peppercorns. Set the chicken on top and pour water over. Bring to a boil, skimming off any foam that rises to the top.

2. Lock the lid in place and bring cooker up to full pressure over high heat. Reduce heat to medium-low, just to maintain even pressure, and cook for 20 minutes for a 3-lb chicken, 5 to 10 minutes longer for a 3.5- to 4-lb bird. Remove from heat and allow pressure to drop naturally. Check to make sure the chicken is very tender and juices run clear. If not, return to full pressure and cook for 3 to 5 minutes longer depending on doneness. Allow pressure to drop naturally.

3. Strain the stock through a fine strainer into another pot and skim off any fat that rises to the top. Reserve 1/2 cup (125 mL) of the stock for the dill cream sauce. Set remaining stock aside. Remove skin from chicken and separate into pieces. Arrange chicken and vegetables on a serving platter and cover loosely with foil. Keep warm in a 200° F (100° C) oven.

4. DILL CREAM SAUCE: In a small saucepan, melt butter over medium heat. Stir in flour and cook for 1 minute. Gradually whisk in the reserved 1/2 cup (125 mL) of stock and cream. Bring to a boil and cook, stirring, for about 5 minutes or until thickened. Stir in dill and paprika. Season to taste with salt and pepper. Keep warm in a sauceboat.

5. Bring remaining stock to a boil and add egg noodles. Reduce heat and simmer for about 5 minutes or just until noodles are tender.

6. To serve, divide soup between 6 deep soup plates. When the soup course is finished, pass the chicken, vegetables and warm dill sauce.

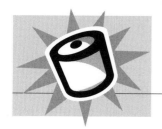

Cajun Chicken and Beer Stew

Serves 8 to 10

This boneless chicken stew takes its inspiration from the spicy cuisine of Cajun country. You'll need a large 7 L pressure cooker to accommodate this stew – halve the recipe if necessary. Mashed potatoes, brown rice or cornbread make perfect accompaniments to this dish.

1 tbsp	salt	15 mL
1 tbsp	garlic powder	15 mL
1 tbsp	cayenne pepper	15 mL
4 lbs	boneless skinless chicken thighs, cut into large chunks	2 kg
1/4 cup	all-purpose flour	50 mL
1/4 cup	olive oil, divided	50 mL
3	cloves garlic, chopped	3
2	stalks celery, chopped	2
1	large onion, chopped	1
1	green pepper, chopped	1
1	red bell pepper, chopped	1
1	green chili pepper, seeded and chopped	1
2	bay leaves	2
2 tsp	dried marjoram	10 mL
1	can (14 oz [398 mL]) tomatoes, puréed	1
1	bottle (12 oz [341 mL]) dark beer (try Big Rock Traditional or Alley Kat Ale if you can find it)	1
1/2 cup	chicken stock	125 mL
1 tbsp	Worcestershire sauce	15 mL
	Salt and freshly ground black pepper to taste	

1. In a small bowl, combine salt, garlic powder and cayenne. Rub chicken all over with 1 tbsp (15 mL) of the spice mixture and let stand at room temperature for 10 minutes.

2. In a plastic bag, combine flour with another 1 tbsp (15 mL) of the spice mixture. Add chicken pieces and shake in spiced flour to coat. Set aside any excess spiced flour.

3. In a pressure cooker, heat 2 tbsp (25 mL) of the oil over medium-high heat. Add chicken in batches and cook until browned. Transfer chicken to bowl and set aside.

4. Reduce heat to medium. Add garlic, celery, onions, green and red bell peppers and chili pepper; sauté for 5 minutes or until onions are tender. Stir in bay leaves, marjoram, tomatoes, beer, stock, Worcestershire and remaining 1 tbsp (15 mL) of spice mixture. Stir in chicken.

5. Lock the lid in place and bring cooker to full pressure over high heat. Reduce heat to medium-low, just to maintain even pressure, and cook for 15 to 20 minutes. Remove from heat and release pressure quickly. Discard bay leaves.

6. Meanwhile, in a skillet, heat remaining 2 tbsp (25 mL) oil over medium heat. Sprinkle in 2 tbsp (25 mL) of the reserved spiced flour, adding extra oil if necessary to create a smooth paste; cook, stirring constantly, until the *roux* turns the color of peanut butter, about 10 minutes. (Be careful – this gets very hot and burns easily.) Whisk a little of the braising liquid from the pressure cooker into skillet. Add this mixture back into the stew and simmer, uncovered, until thick. Season to taste with salt and pepper.

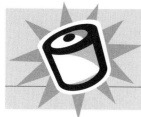

Coq Au Vin

Serves 6

This is a classic French country stew, perfect to serve over noodles or boiled potatoes. It's elegant enough for company but easy enough for every day. Don't skip the cognac – it adds authenticity to this hearty bistro fare.

TIP

To remove skins from pearl onions, submerge them in boiling water for a few minutes, then run under cold water and peel.

2	sprigs thyme	2
1	sprig parsley	1
1	bay leaf	1
3 1/2 lbs	boneless skinless chicken pieces (breasts and thighs)	1.75 kg
4	slices double-smoked bacon, chopped	4
1 tbsp	olive oil (approximate)	15 mL
10	pearl onions or shallots, peeled (see Tip, at left)	10
2	cloves garlic, minced	2
2	stalks celery, sliced	2
1	carrot, grated	1
2 cups	dry red wine	500 mL
1/4 cup	cognac	50 mL
8 oz	white mushrooms, halved (or quartered, if large)	250 g
2 tbsp	cornstarch dissolved in 2 tbsp (25 mL) water	25 mL
3 tbsp	chopped parsley	45 mL
	Salt and freshly ground black pepper	

1. Using kitchen string, tie thyme, parsley and bay leaf into a *bouquet garni*. Set aside.

2. In a pressure cooker over medium-high heat, sauté bacon until starting to crisp. Add chicken pieces in batches and cook until brown, adding more olive oil if necessary to prevent chicken from sticking. Transfer to a bowl and set aside. Reduce heat to medium. Add onions and garlic; sauté until onions start to brown. Stir in celery, carrot, wine, cognac, mushrooms, *bouquet garni*, chicken, bacon and any accumulated juices.

3. Lock the lid in place and bring cooker up to full pressure over high heat. Reduce heat to medium-low, just to maintain even pressure, and cook for 10 to 12 minutes. Remove from heat and release pressure quickly.

4. Whisk cornstarch mixture into stew; cook over medium heat until juices are thick and glossy. Discard the *bouquet garni*. Stir in parsley and season to taste with salt and pepper. Serve chicken over wide egg noodles or surrounded by boiled new potatoes, sprinkled with additional chopped parsley.

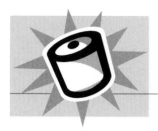

Chicken with Chorizo Sausage and Rice

Serves 4

This is a South American-style rice dish, reminiscent of Spanish paella or jambalaya. The timing is critical here – after 10 minutes under pressure, and another 5 minutes of steaming, all of the liquid should be absorbed and the rice should be fluffy.

3 cups	chicken stock	750 mL
2	threads saffron, crushed	2
2 lbs	boneless skinless chicken thighs, cut into 2-inch (5 cm) chunks	1 kg
2 tbsp	olive oil	25 mL
2	cloves garlic, minced	2
1	onion, chopped	1
1	green pepper, chopped	1
1	red bell pepper, chopped	1
4 to 8 oz	chorizo or other spicy sausage, chopped (or crumbled if fresh)	125 to 250 g
2	plum tomatoes, seeded and chopped	2
1 3/4 cups	long grain rice	425 mL
1 cup	frozen peas, thawed	250 mL
2 tbsp	chopped parsley	25 mL

1. In a bowl stir together stock and saffron; set aside to infuse.
2. In a pressure cooker, heat oil over medium-high heat. Add chicken in batches and cook until browned. Remove chicken to a bowl and set aside.
3. Reduce heat to medium. Add garlic, onion, green and red peppers; sauté for 5 minutes or until onion is softened. Stir in sausage, rice and tomatoes; sauté for another 3 minutes. Arrange browned chicken on top of rice and pour stock mixture over top.
4. Lock the lid in place and bring cooker up to full pressure over high heat. Reduce heat to medium-low, just to maintain even pressure, and cook for 10 minutes. Remove from heat and allow pressure to drop naturally for 5 minutes. Release any remaining pressure quickly. Stir in peas and sprinkle with parsley.

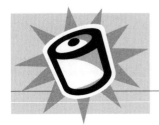

Turkey with Prunes and Armagnac

Serves 4 to 6

This dish is inspired by the classic combination of rabbit, Agen prunes and brandy, which is popular in the southwestern part of France. Turkey makes a great substitute but, by all means, try this recipe with rabbit if it is available. The rich, dark sauce in this dish also works well with chicken or duck. Serve it over spaetzle (fresh dumplings), noodles or rice.

TIP

If you decide to use duck in this recipe, precook it in the pressure cooker to remove the fat before adding it to the sauce. This eliminates the browning step used for turkey. Just place a trivet or steamer basket in cooker and add 3 cups (750 mL) water. Place 3 lbs (1.5 kg) duck legs in the cooker and steam under full pressure for 10 minutes. Drain, remove trivet, then add remaining ingredients; cook for 10 minutes longer.

3 lbs	boneless skinless turkey thighs or breast, cut into 8 to 10 pieces	1.5 kg
1/4 cup	all-purpose flour	50 mL
1/2 tsp	salt	2 mL
1/4 tsp	freshly ground black pepper	1 mL
3 tbsp	olive oil	45 mL
2 oz	finely diced bacon	50 g
4	carrots, sliced	4
2	cloves garlic, minced	2
2 tsp	chopped thyme	10 mL
1	onion, slivered	1
1	stalk celery, minced	1
1 cup	chopped pitted prunes	250 mL
1 cup	dry red wine	250 mL
2 tbsp	honey	25 mL
1/3 cup	Armagnac or other brandy	75 mL
1/2 cup	water *or* chicken stock	125 mL

1. In a plastic bag, combine flour with salt and pepper. Add turkey pieces and toss to coat. In a pressure cooker, heat oil over medium heat. Add bacon and cook, stirring, until bacon begins to render its fat. Add turkey in batches and cook until browned. Transfer turkey to a bowl and set aside.

2. Add carrots, garlic, thyme, onion and celery to cooker; sauté for 2 minutes. Add cooked turkey and top with prunes. In a bowl combine wine, honey, brandy and water; pour over turkey.

3. Lock the lid in place and bring cooker up to full pressure over high heat. Reduce heat to medium-low, just to maintain even pressure, and cook for 10 minutes. Remove from heat and release pressure quickly.

4. Transfer turkey to a warmed deep platter. If desired, simmer sauce to reduce and thicken; spoon over turkey and serve.

Moroccan Lemon Chicken Tagine with Couscous

Serves 4 to 6

A tagine is a Moroccan stew. This version replaces the traditional preserved lemons (lemons cured in salt) with lemon zest and juice.

2 lbs	boneless skinless chicken breasts, each halved crosswise	1 kg
2 tbsp	butter	25 mL
1 tbsp	extra virgin olive oil	15 mL
2	large onions, finely chopped	2
2	cloves garlic, minced	2
2 tsp	minced ginger root	10 mL
1 tsp	ground cumin	5 mL
1/2 tsp	crumbled saffron threads	2 mL
2 cups	chicken stock	500 mL
	Zest of 1 large lemon, minced	
	Juice of 1 large lemon (about 1/4 cup [50 mL])	
2 tbsp	honey	25 mL
12	large green olives, pitted	12
2 tbsp	cornstarch dissolved in 2 tbsp (25 mL) water	25 mL
2 tbsp	chopped Italian parsley	25 mL
	Salt and freshly ground black pepper to taste	
2 cups	couscous	500 mL
2 1/4 cups	chicken stock	300 mL

1. In a pressure cooker, heat butter and oil over medium heat. Add chicken in batches and cook until browned, transferring cooked pieces to a bowl. Once all the chicken is browned, return it to the cooker. Add onion, garlic and ginger; sauté for 5 minutes. Stir in saffron, cumin, stock and half of the lemon zest. Add lemon juice and honey.

2. Lock the lid in place and bring cooker up to full pressure over high heat. Reduce heat to medium-low, just to maintain even pressure, and cook for 8 minutes. Remove from heat and release pressure quickly.

3. Stir in olives and remaining lemon zest. Whisk in cornstarch mixture; simmer until sauce is syrupy and smooth. Stir in parsley; season to taste with salt and pepper.

4. Meanwhile, in a saucepan bring chicken stock to a boil; stir in the couscous, cover and remove from heat; let stand for 5 minutes. Fluff couscous with a fork and pile it on a large serving platter, making a well in the center. Arrange chicken pieces in the center, and spoon sauce over and around.

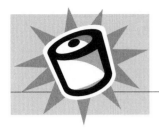

Speedy Dijon Chicken

Serves 4

This almost-instant chicken dish is ideal for a weekday family meal, but elegant enough to impress dinner guests.

Crème fraîche is a thickened heavy cream – easy to make with a little sour cream or yogurt and a container of whipping (35%) cream. Just mix 2 cups (500 mL) whipping cream with 1/2 cup (125 mL) sour cream and let stand, covered, at room temperature for 12 hours. When the mixture is nicely thickened, you can store it in the refrigerator for up to 2 weeks. *Crème fraîche* also makes a lovely dessert topping.

2 lbs	boneless skinless chicken breasts	1 kg
1 tbsp	olive oil	15 mL
1	small onion, minced	1
3 tbsp	Dijon mustard	45 mL
1 tbsp	grainy mustard	15 mL
1 tbsp	honey	15 mL
1/2 cup	chicken stock	125 mL
1/4 cup	dry white wine *or* apple juice	50 mL
1/2 cup	sour cream or *crème fraîche* (see note, at left)	125 mL
2 tbsp	all-purpose flour	25 mL
	Chopped fresh herbs for garnish	

1. In a pressure cooker, heat oil over medium-high heat. Add chicken in batches and cook for about 5 minutes or until browned.

2. In a small bowl, whisk together Dijon mustard, grainy mustard and honey; gradually whisk in stock and wine. Pour over the chicken.

3. Lock the lid in place and bring cooker up to full pressure over high heat. Reduce heat to medium-low, just to maintain even pressure, and cook chicken for 8 minutes. Remove from heat and release pressure quickly.

4. Transfer chicken to a serving platter and tent with foil to keep warm. In a small bowl, whisk sour cream with flour; whisk into cooker. Simmer over low heat for 2 to 3 minutes or until thickened. Pour sauce over chicken and garnish with fresh herbs. Serve with steamed broccoli and wild rice or steamed new potatoes.

WHOLE 'ROASTED' CHICKEN WITH LEMON, GARLIC AND HERBS (PAGE 65) ➤

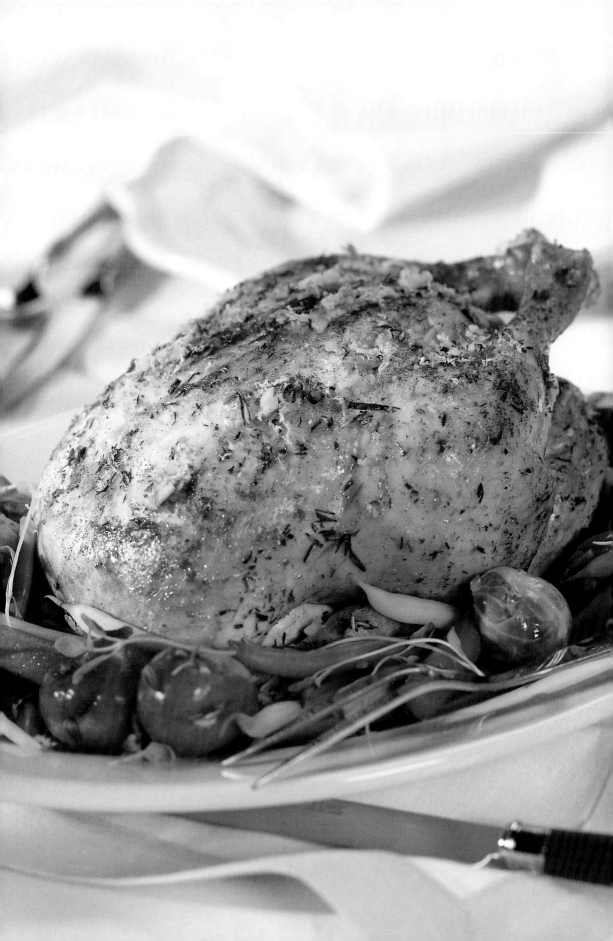

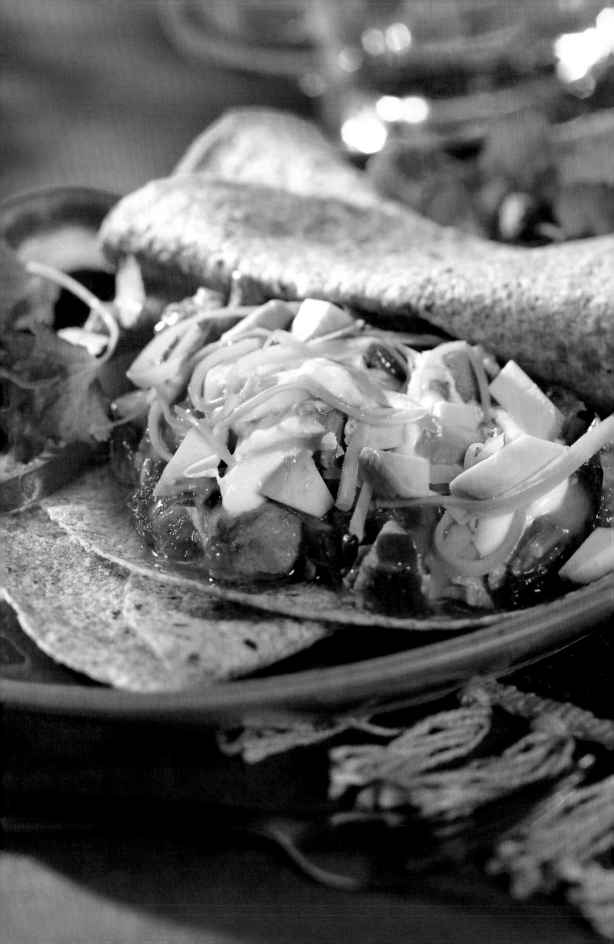

Whole 'Roasted' Chicken with Lemon, Garlic and Herbs

Serves 4

This braised bird comes out meltingly tender and infused with the flavors of lemon, garlic, rosemary and thyme. You can crisp the skin by putting it into a hot (450° F [220° C]) preheated oven for 10 to 15 minutes, or simply remove the skin for serving. This chicken is also wonderful cold – the perfect way to create flavorful, moist chicken for your next picnic or salad.

1	chicken, about 3 lbs (1.5 kg) or a size that will fit comfortably into your pressure cooker	1
4	cloves garlic, minced	4
1 tbsp	chopped thyme	15 mL
1 tbsp	chopped rosemary	15 mL
	Zest of 1 lemon, minced	
	Juice of 1 lemon	
2 tbsp	olive oil	25 mL
2 cups	chicken stock	500 mL
	Freshly ground black pepper	
2 tbsp	cornstarch dissolved in 1 tbsp (15 mL) water	25 mL

1. In a small bowl, combine garlic, thyme and rosemary; rub half of the mixture inside chicken. Rub the inside with 1 tbsp (15 mL) of the lemon juice and 1 tsp (5 mL) of the lemon zest.

2. In a pressure cooker, heat oil over high heat. Add chicken and brown on all sides. Pour in stock and remaining lemon juice; sprinkle with remaining garlic mixture.

3. Lock the lid in place and bring cooker up to full pressure over high heat. Reduce heat to medium-low, just to maintain even pressure, and cook for 25 to 30 minutes. Remove from heat and release pressure quickly. Chicken should be tender, with an internal temperature of 170° F (75° C). If not, return cooker to full pressure and cook for 5 minutes or longer, depending on doneness. Remove from heat and release pressure quickly.

4. Transfer chicken to a carving board and tent with foil to keep warm. Pour cooking juices into a glass measuring cup; skim off any fat. Return liquid to cooker and bring to a boil. Whisk in cornstarch mixture and cook, stirring, for about 3 minutes or until gravy is thickened. Season to taste with pepper and stir in remaining 1 tsp (5 mL) lemon zest. Carve chicken from the bone and serve with gravy (remove skin if desired).

◄ PORK WRAPS WITH GREEN TOMATOES AND ANCHO CHILIES (PAGE 78)

Jamaican Chicken Fricassee

Serves 4 to 6

Start the chicken marinating the night before you plan to serve this savory, island-inspired dish, or at least get it going in the morning before you head off to work.

Scotch bonnet chilies are the hottest type you can buy. Substitute jalapeño or serrano chilies, but up the amount to give this dish the right amount of spicy flavor. Or pass one of those searing Jamaican hot sauces now available for those who like their chicken really smokin'.

MARINADE

	Juice of 1 lime	
2	cloves garlic	2
2 tsp	fresh thyme leaves	10 mL
1	Scotch bonnet chili	1
1 tbsp	Worcestershire sauce	15 mL
1 tsp	whole or ground allspice	5 mL
	Salt and freshly ground black pepper	
3 lbs	boneless skinless chicken thighs *or* 4 lbs (2 kg) chicken pieces, skin removed	1.5 kg
1 tbsp	vegetable oil	15 mL
1 tbsp	packed dark brown sugar	15 mL
1	onion, minced	1
3	tomatoes, peeled and chopped	3
1 cup	chicken stock	250 mL
1	bay leaf	1
1 tsp	hot pepper sauce (or to taste)	5 mL
5	green onions, minced	5
	Chopped fresh parsley	

1. MARINADE: In a food processor or mini-chopper, purée lime juice, garlic, thyme, Scotch bonnet, Worcestershire and allspice. In a large shallow glass dish, pour marinade over chicken pieces and turn to coat well. Cover and refrigerate for at least 2 hours or overnight. Drain, reserving marinade.

2. In a pressure cooker, heat oil and sugar over medium-high heat; cook, stirring, until sugar is melted. Add chicken pieces in batches and cook, turning frequently, for about 10 minutes or until browned. Transfer to a bowl and set aside.

3. Reduce heat to medium. Add onion and sauté for 5 minutes. Stir in reserved marinade, tomatoes, stock, bay leaf and hot pepper sauce. Return chicken to the cooker with any accumulated juices.

4. Lock the lid in place and bring cooker up to full pressure over high heat. Reduce heat to medium-low, just to maintain even pressure, and cook for 10 minutes. Remove from heat and release pressure quickly. Discard bay leaf.

5. Transfer chicken to a warmed deep serving platter. Bring braising liquid to a boil and reduce until thickened to desired consistency. Pour sauce over chicken and garnish with green onions and parsley.

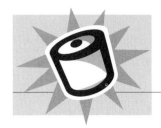

Chicken Thighs with Curry Sauce and Couscous

Serves 6

Garam masala is an Indian spice mixture that you can find in the Asian section of most large supermarkets.

TIP

If you're pressed for time, use 2 tbsp (25 mL) curry paste to replace the minced garlic, chili powder, cayenne, coriander, cumin and turmeric.

2 tbsp	butter	25 mL
1	large onion, finely chopped	1
2	cloves garlic, minced	2
1 tsp	chili powder	5 mL
1/2 tsp	cayenne pepper	2 mL
2 tsp	ground coriander	10 mL
1 tsp	ground cumin	5 mL
1 tsp	turmeric	5 mL
1 cup	chopped plum tomatoes	250 mL
2 lbs	boneless skinless chicken thighs, cut into 1-inch (2.5 cm) cubes	1 kg
	Juice of 1 lemon	
1/2 tsp	salt	2 mL
1/2 cup	chicken stock	125 mL
2 tsp	garam masala	10 mL
1	small red bell pepper, cut into slivers	1
1	small zucchini, cut into matchstick strips	1
1 cup	couscous	250 mL
1/4 cup	chopped cilantro	50 mL
	Salt to taste	

1. In a pressure cooker, melt butter over medium heat. Add garlic and onion; cook until softened. Add chili powder, cayenne, coriander, cumin, turmeric and tomatoes; sauté until tomatoes are soft. Add chicken and sprinkle with lemon juice and salt. Pour in stock.

2. Lock the lid in place and bring cooker up to full pressure over high heat. Reduce heat to medium-low, just to maintain even pressure, and cook for 12 minutes. Remove from heat and release pressure quickly.

3. Stir in garam masala, red pepper, zucchini strips and couscous. Return lid to cooker (do not lock into place) or cover with another pot lid and let stand for 5 minutes. Fluff couscous with a fork. Stir in cilantro and season to taste with salt. Serve immediately.

Chicken in Creamy Mushroom Sauce

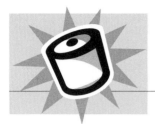

Serves 4

Just like that old family favorite – only faster. (And no canned soup!) Serve the chicken and sauce over pasta or mashed potatoes.

2 tbsp	butter	25 mL
4	boneless skinless chicken breasts	4
2 cups	sliced mushrooms	500 mL
1	onion, chopped	1
1	clove garlic, minced	1
1 cup	chicken stock	250 mL
2 tbsp	sherry	25 mL
1 tsp	Dijon mustard	5 mL
1/3 cup	whipping (35%) cream	75 mL
	Salt and freshly ground black pepper to taste	

1. In a pressure cooker, melt butter over medium-high heat. Add chicken in batches and sauté until lightly browned. Transfer browned chicken to a bowl. Set aside.

2. Add mushrooms, onion and garlic to cooker; sauté until fragrant and beginning to brown. Place browned chicken on top of vegetables. Pour in stock and sherry.

3. Lock the lid in place and bring cooker up to full pressure over high heat. Reduce heat to medium-low, just to maintain even pressure, and cook for 5 minutes. Remove from heat and release pressure quickly.

4. Transfer chicken to a warm platter. Whisk mustard and cream into cooker; bring to a boil and cook for 3 minutes or until reduced and thickened. Season sauce to taste with salt and pepper; pour over the chicken. Serve with pasta or mashed potatoes.

Meat

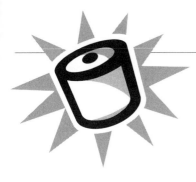

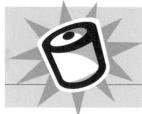

Perfect Pot Roast

Serves 6

Use beef rump or round roast in this flavorful pot roast recipe, a classic comfort food. You can also substitute bison, a popular new red meat which is ultra-lean and raised without growth hormones and antibiotics. The braising makes it tender and the puréed vegetables add richness to the gravy without extra fat. And it's done in less than an hour!

1	3 1/2 lb (1.75 kg) beef or bison braising roast	1
1/4 cup	all-purpose flour	50 mL
1/2 tsp	salt	2 mL
1/4 tsp	freshly ground black pepper	1 mL
3 tbsp	vegetable oil *or* olive oil	45 mL
1	large tomato, chopped	1
1 cup	diced onions	250 mL
1 cup	diced carrots	250 mL
1/2 cup	diced celery	125 mL
1 cup	beef stock	250 mL
1 cup	dry red wine	250 mL
2 tbsp	all-purpose flour whisked with 2 tbsp (25 mL) cold water	25 mL
1 lb	wide egg noodles, cooked and tossed with butter *or* steamed new potatoes	500 g
	Minced fresh thyme or oregano to taste	

1. In a plastic bag, combine 1/4 cup (50 mL) flour with salt and pepper. Add roast and shake to coat all sides with flour. Discard excess flour mixture.

2. In a pressure cooker, heat oil over medium-high heat and brown roast well on all sides. Transfer to plate. Set aside.

3. Add tomato, onions, carrots and celery to pan; sauté until lightly browned. Place roast on top of vegetables. Pour in stock and wine.

4. Lock the lid in place and bring cooker up to full pressure over high heat. Reduce heat to medium-low, just to maintain even pressure, and cook for 45 minutes. Remove from heat and release pressure quickly.

5. Transfer roast to a platter and tent with foil to keep warm. In a blender or food processor, purée vegetables and stock. Return to pot and slowly whisk in flour mixture. Bring to a boil; reduce heat and simmer until gravy is thickened, about 5 minutes. Season gravy with salt and pepper to taste. Season to taste with thyme or oregano. Arrange egg noodles or potatoes around roast on platter and drizzle with gravy.

Barbecue Beef on a Bun

Serves 8

This is a perfect meal for any summer party crowd. It can be precooked quickly in the pressure cooker early in the day, then finished on the barbecue during the party. Set out some old washtubs filled with beer and ice, and serve some coleslaw and potato salad on the side for a real cowboy experience. Yee-Ha!

1	beef brisket, about 3 lbs (1.5 kg)	1
3	cloves garlic, minced	3
1	large onion, minced	1
1	chipotle chili in adobo, chopped *or* 1 jalapeño chili, chopped and 1 tsp (5 mL) liquid smoke	1
1/2 cup	packed brown sugar	125 mL
1	bottle (12 oz [341 mL]) dark beer	1
1 cup	ketchup	250 mL
2 tbsp	Dijon mustard	25 mL
1 tbsp	chili powder	15 mL
1 tbsp	dried basil	15 mL
1 tsp	ground cumin	5 mL
	Worcestershire sauce to taste	
	Salt and freshly ground black pepper	
	Crusty onion rolls	

1. Trim fat from brisket and roll into an evenly-shaped roast, tying at intervals. Season with salt and freshly ground black pepper. Place brisket in pressure cooker.

2. In a bowl, whisk together garlic, onion, chipotle, brown sugar, beer, ketchup, mustard, chili powder, basil, cumin and Worcestershire sauce; pour over top of meat.

3. Lock the lid in place and bring cooker up to full pressure over high heat. Reduce heat to medium-low, just to maintain even pressure, and cook for 45 minutes. Remove from heat and release pressure quickly. Transfer brisket to a plate. Cover and refrigerate. Skim as much fat from the sauce as possible and simmer for 30 minutes to reduce and thicken. Set aside.

4. Just before serving, place roast on a preheated barbecue over medium-low heat and cook for 15 minutes until slightly charred and smoky, turning frequently.

5. Slice brisket thinly, or shred; mix in some of the reserved barbecue sauce and pile on a bun. You can also make this in advance and reheat the meat in the sauce. Serve with beans, coleslaw and potato salad or baked potatoes on the side.

Spicy Beef and Beer Stew

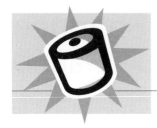

Serves 8 to 10

Sweet, spicy and savory, this is beef stew with an attitude. Add a crusty loaf of French bread and it's a meal.

2	cloves garlic, minced	2
1/4 cup	packed brown sugar	50 mL
1 tsp	ground cumin	5 mL
1 tsp	salt	5 mL
1/2 tsp	freshly ground black pepper	2 mL
1/4 tsp	ground cinnamon	1 mL
5 lbs	boneless beef chuck steak, cut into large chunks	2.5 kg
2 tbsp	vegetable oil	25 mL
2	large onions, cut into wedges	2
1	green pepper, cut into chunks	1
1	bottle (12 oz [341 mL]) dark beer	1
2	tomatoes, diced *or* 3 tbsp [45 mL] tomato paste	2
1 tsp	red pepper flakes	5 mL
10	small new potatoes, halved	10
16	baby carrots	16
2 tbsp	all-purpose flour whisked with 2 tbsp (25 mL) cold water (optional)	25 mL

1. In a large bowl, combine garlic, 1 tbsp (15 mL) of the sugar, cumin, salt, pepper and cinnamon. Add beef cubes and stir to coat. Cover and refrigerate for 1 hour.

2. In a pressure cooker, heat oil over medium-high heat; brown meat, in batches. Return browned meat to cooker. Add onion and green pepper; sauté for 5 minutes. In a bowl combine beer, diced tomato, pepper flakes and remaining brown sugar; pour into cooker. Stir in potatoes and carrots.

3. Lock the lid in place and bring cooker up to full pressure over high heat. Reduce the heat to medium-low, just to maintain even pressure, and cook for 35 minutes. Remove from heat and release pressure quickly.

4. If desired, whisk in flour mixture and bring to a boil; reduce heat and simmer for about 5 minutes or until thickened.

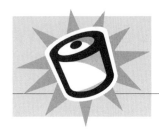

Beef Shortribs in Barbecue Sauce

Serves 4

This is the best – and fastest – way to cook lean beef shortribs or big meaty side ribs. These cuts are actually more flavorful than tender cuts such as T-bone steaks; it's a revelation when you can make them tender, too.

TIP

The suace in this recipe is also a good for marinating flank steak before barbecuing.

If you can't buy boneless beef short ribs, use 4 lbs (2 kg) bone-in ribs and remove the bones yourself or have your butcher de-bone them.

2 to 3 lbs	boneless beef short ribs *or* big beef side ribs	1 to 1.5 kg
1 tbsp	vegetable oil	15 mL
2	cloves garlic, minced	2
1	onion, minced	1
1/4 cup	packed brown sugar	50 mL
1 tsp	freshly ground black pepper	5 mL
1	can (14 oz [398 mL]) tomato sauce	1
1/2 cup	chili sauce	125 mL
1/2 cup	strong coffee	125 mL
1/2 cup	beef stock	125 mL
1 tbsp	Worcestershire sauce	15 mL
1 tbsp	molasses	15 mL
1 tsp	liquid smoke	5 mL
1 tsp	hot pepper sauce	5 mL

1. In a pressure cooker, heat oil over medium-high heat. Add ribs in batches and cook for about 15 minutes or until browned. Transfer ribs to a bowl; set aside. Discard any excess fat.

2. Reduce heat to medium. Add garlic and onion; sauté for about 3 minutes until soft. Add sugar, pepper, tomato sauce, chili sauce, coffee, stock, Worcestershire, molasses, liquid smoke and hot pepper sauce; simmer for 15 minutes, scraping up any browned bits from bottom of cooker. Return ribs to cooker along with any accumulated juices.

3. Lock the lid in place and bring cooker up to low pressure over medium-high heat. Reduce heat to medium-low, just to maintain even pressure, and cook for 25 minutes. Remove from heat and release pressure quickly.

4. Simmer, uncovered, for another 10 minutes, basting often, until ribs are glazed and sauce is thickened. Serve ribs along with lots of horseradish, beans and baked potatoes.

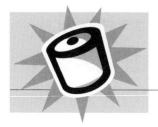

Pork Loin Chops with Red Cabbage and Apples

Serves 4

The red cabbage and apples make a colorful and healthful backdrop for tender pork loin chops. The faintly sweet braising liquid makes a wonderful drizzle when you cook it down to a thick syrup.

2 tbsp	olive oil	25 mL
4	lean center-cut pork loin chops, about 1 inch (2.5 cm) thick, trimmed of visible fat	4
3 tbsp	butter	45 mL
1	red onion, halved and slivered	1
1 lb	red cabbage, shredded	500 g
1/2 cup	chicken stock	125 mL
1/2 cup	dry white wine	125 mL
1	bay leaf	1
1/2 tsp	salt	2 mL
1/8 tsp	freshly ground black pepper	0.5 mL
2	Granny Smith apples, peeled, cored and cut into wedges	2

1. In a pressure cooker, heat oil over medium-high heat. Add pork chops and cook about 2 minutes per side or until browned. Transfer to a plate. Set aside.

2. Melt butter in cooker and sauté red onion for 5 minutes, until soft and beginning to brown. Stir in cabbage to coat with butter. Add stock, wine, bay leaf, salt, pepper and apples. Place pork chops on top.

3. Lock the lid in place and bring cooker up to full pressure over medium-high heat. Reduce heat to medium-low, just to maintain even pressure, and cook for 14 minutes. Remove from heat and release pressure quickly. Discard bay leaf.

4. Using a slotted spoon, transfer pork chops and cabbage to a platter with cabbage on the bottom and pork on top. Bring braising liquid to boil over high heat; cook until reduced and thickened. Drizzle sauce over pork and cabbage; season with additional pepper to taste.

Pork Wraps with Green Tomatoes and Ancho Chilies

Serves 6

This is a traditional Mexican stew, made with tart, green tomatillos, a vegetable that resembles a small green tomato in a papery husk. You can substitute unripe, green tomatoes in the fall, or even use regular tomatoes with an added 1 tbsp (15 mL) lemon juice for tartness.

Ancho or pasilla chilies are medium-hot dried chilies; fresh banana or Hungarian peppers are the closest substitute.

2 tbsp	olive oil	25 mL
1 1/2 lbs	pork shoulder, fat removed, cut into chunks	750 g
4	cloves garlic, minced	4
1 tsp	salt	5 mL
1	large onion, chopped	1
1 cup	green tomatoes *or* chopped tomatillos *or* 1 (10 oz [284 mL]) can tomatillos	250 mL
1 cup	chopped ripe tomatoes	250 mL
1 cup	dark beer	250 mL
1/2 cup	orange juice	125 mL
1	jalapeño pepper, seeded and chopped	1
2	dried ancho or pasilla chilies, seeded and crumbled	2
1 tsp	ground cumin	5 mL
2 tbsp	all-purpose flour whisked with 2 tbsp (25 mL) cold water	25 mL
1/2 cup	chopped cilantro (about half a bunch)	125 mL
1 1/2 cups	frozen corn kernels, thawed	375 mL
12	large whole wheat tortillas *or* hot cooked brown rice	12
	Garnishes: sliced avocado, grated cheddar and sour cream	

1. In a pressure cooker, heat oil over medium-high heat. Add pork in batches and cook until browned. Transfer to a bowl. Set aside.

2. Reduce heat to medium. Add garlic and sauté until fragrant. Season with salt. Add onions and sauté for about 10 minutes or until they start to brown. Return pork to cooker; add tomatillos, tomatoes, beer, orange juice, jalapeño pepper, dried chilies and cumin.

3. Lock lid in place and bring cooker up to full pressure over high heat. Reduce heat to medium-low, just to maintain even pressure, and cook for 20 minutes. Remove from heat and release pressure quickly.

4. Whisk in flour mixture and cook, stirring, for 5 minutes or until thickened. Add corn and cook for 2 minutes longer. Stir in cilantro and serve immediately wrapped in tortillas with garnishes, or over rice.

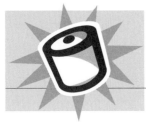

Kansas City Pulled Pork Butt

Serves 6 to 8

Pulled pork is traditionally slow-cooked in a smoker, then shredded and served on a bun with coleslaw.

This isn't exactly what you'd find in Kansas (purists would cringe), but it's a reasonable facsimile, and makes a delicious, tender shredded pork to pile on a sandwich. The ballpark mustard slather and spices are traditional, though. Don't be tempted to substitute Dijon, it's not sugary enough for this recipe. Try it – you'll like it.

TIP

Instead of simmering the braising liquid, thicken with 1 tbsp (15 mL) cornstarch dissolved in 1 tbsp (15 mL) cold water. Whisk into liquid and simmer for about 3 minutes or until thickened.

RACK OR TRIVET TO FIT BOTTOM OF PRESSURE COOKER

1	2-lb (1 kg) boneless pork shoulder roast, tied	1
1 tbsp	liquid smoke	15 mL
1/4 cup	prepared mustard	50 mL

DRY RUB

2 tbsp	granulated sugar	25 mL
2 tbsp	paprika	25 mL
1 tbsp	packed brown sugar	15 mL
1 tbsp	ground cumin	15 mL
1 tbsp	chili powder	15 mL
1 tbsp	freshly ground black pepper	15 mL
1 tsp	salt	5 mL
1 tsp	cayenne pepper	5 mL
1/4 tsp	ground ginger	1 mL
1/4 tsp	ground allspice	1 mL
1/4 tsp	ground cloves	1 mL
3 tbsp	packed brown sugar	45 mL
1/2 tsp	salt	2 mL
1 cup	water	250 mL
1/2 cup	beer	125 mL
1/4 cup	tomato paste	50 mL
2 tbsp	vinegar	25 mL
1 tsp	liquid smoke	15 mL
8	crusty whole wheat buns	8
	Coleslaw	

1. Drizzle surface of meat with 1 tbsp (15 mL) liquid smoke and rub to coat well, making sure to get some into the inside surfaces, where the roast is rolled and tied. Let stand for 10 minutes. Spread mustard over pork.

2. DRY RUB: In a small bowl, combine granulated sugar, paprika, brown sugar, cumin, chili powder, pepper, salt, cayenne, ginger, allspice and cloves. Sprinkle mixture generously over all surfaces of the pork. Let stand at room temperature until the rub gets nice and tacky, about 10 minutes. (This will form a crust on the meat as it cooks.)

3. In a pressure cooker, whisk together brown sugar, salt, water, beer, tomato paste, vinegar and liquid smoke. Set rack in cooker and place pork on top.

4. Lock the lid in place and bring cooker up to full pressure over high heat. Reduce heat to medium-low, just to maintain even pressure, and cook for 1 1/2 hours. Remove from heat and allow pressure to drop naturally. The internal temperature should be at least 170° F (75° C) and the pork should be tender enough to shred. If not, return to full pressure and cook for 5 to 10 minutes longer.

5. Transfer pork to a bowl and let cool slightly. Using two forks, shred the meat. Discard any excess fat. Bring braising liquid to a boil; reduce heat and simmer until reduced and slightly thickened. Drizzle some of the sauce over the pork and toss well to combine. Serve pulled pork piled on buns with coleslaw on top and remaining sauce on the side.

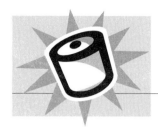

Lamb Rogan Josh

Serves 4 to 6

This is a classic Indian curry that's perfect for a party. Use lean lamb (or substitute beef) and marinate overnight for layers of deep, rich flavor. Serve the tender lamb curry with golden INDIAN RICE PILAU, seasoned with cinnamon, turmeric and cardamom (see recipe, page 147).

2 lbs	lean lamb shoulder, trimmed and cut into chunks	1 kg
1/2 cup	plain yogurt	125 mL
4	green cardamom pods	4
1	small cinnamon stick *or* 1/2 tsp (2 mL) ground cinnamon	1
2 tsp	paprika	10 mL
1 tsp	turmeric	5 mL
1 tsp	ground coriander	5 mL
1 tsp	ground cumin	5 mL
1/2 tsp	cayenne pepper	2 mL
2 tsp	garam masala	10 mL
2 cups	canned tomatoes	500 mL
2	cloves garlic, peeled	2
1	large onion, chopped	1
1	2-inch (5 cm) piece ginger root	1
3 tbsp	vegetable oil	45 mL
1 cup	water	250 mL
2 tbsp	chopped cilantro	25 mL
	Cilantro springs for garnish	

1. In a bowl or zippered plastic bag, toss lamb with yogurt. In a blender or spice grinder, pulverize whole cardamom and cinnamon. Add to lamb mixture with paprika, turmeric, coriander, cumin and cayenne. Cover and refrigerate overnight.

2. In a food processor, combine garam masala, tomatoes, garlic, onion and ginger; purée until smooth.

3. In a pressure cooker, heat oil over medium heat. Add tomato mixture and cook for 5 minutes. Stir in lamb and marinade. Stir in water.

4. Lock the lid in place and bring cooker up to full pressure over medium-high heat. Reduce heat to medium-low, just to maintain even pressure, and cook for 20 minutes. Remove from heat and release pressure quickly. The lamb should be fork tender. If not, return to full pressure and cook for another 5 minutes. Release pressure quickly.

5. Remove lid and bring to boil. Reduce heat and simmer curry until nicely thickened. Stir in cilantro just before serving. Garnish with cilantro sprigs.

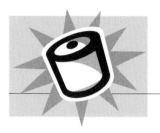

Creamy Pork Goulash with Porcini Mushrooms

Serves 6

Serve this goulash with plenty of wide egg noodles to soak up all of the delicious, creamy sauce. For added zip, try it with a black pepper pasta.

2 lbs	boneless pork shoulder roast or pork steaks, trimmed and cubed	1 kg
1 tbsp	olive oil	15 mL
1	large onion, sliced	1
2	cloves garlic, minced	2
1	red or yellow bell pepper, seeded and sliced	1
1	can (10 oz [284 mL]) chicken broth, undiluted	1
3/4 cup	dry white wine	175 mL
1 oz	dried porcini mushrooms	30 g
1	tomato, seeded and chopped	1
1 tsp	sweet Spanish paprika	5 mL
6	extra-large green olives (preferably stuffed with garlic), sliced	6
3 tbsp	all-purpose flour	45 mL
1/4 cup	sour cream	50 mL
1 lb	wide egg noodles	500 g
	Chopped parsley	

1. In a pressure cooker, heat oil over medium-high heat. Add pork in batches and cook until browned. Transfer to a bowl. Set aside.

2. Reduce heat to medium. Add onion and sauté until it starts to brown. Stir in garlic and red pepper; sauté for 2 minutes. Stir in broth, wine, mushrooms, tomato, paprika and pork with any accumulated juices.

3. Lock the lid in place and bring cooker up to full pressure over high heat. Reduce heat to medium-low, just to maintain even pressure, and cook for 12 minutes. Remove from heat and release pressure quickly. Stir in olives.

4. In a small bowl, whisk flour together with sour cream; whisk into to the stew. Simmer, stirring, for about 5 minutes until thickened. Meanwhile, in a large pot of boiling salted water, cook egg noodles until almost tender. Drain and add to stew; cook for about 10 minutes longer or until noodles are tender. Transfer goulash to a deep platter and garnish with parsley.

Spanish Lamb Stew Braised in Rioja

Serves 4

This is a wonderful way to use an inexpensive cut of lamb. Start this dish the day before you plan to serve it, so that the meat has plenty of time to marinate.

3 lbs	lamb shoulder, cut into 2-inch (5 cm) chunks	1.5 kg
1 cup	Rioja or other dry, fruity red wine, divided	250 mL
5	cloves garlic, minced, divided	5
	Leaves from 1 sprig of rosemary, minced	
1/4 cup	all-purpose flour	50 mL
1/2 tsp	salt	2 mL
1/4 tsp	freshly ground black pepper	1 mL
3 tbsp	olive oil	45 mL
1	large onion, chopped	1
1 tbsp	sweet Spanish or Hungarian paprika	15 mL
1	bay leaf	1
1	can (14 oz [398 mL]) plum tomatoes, chopped	1
1/2 cup	beef stock *or* chicken stock	125 mL
1/2 cup	roasted red pepper, chopped	125 mL

1. In a zippered plastic bag, combine lamb, 1/2 cup (125 mL) of wine, 3 cloves of the garlic and rosemary; refrigerate overnight.

2. Drain lamb, reserving marinade. Pat dry with paper towels. In a large bowl, toss lamb with salt and pepper, then with flour, coating well; discard excess flour. In a pressure cooker, heat oil over medium-high heat. Add lamb in batches and cook until browned.

3. Return browned lamb to cooker. Add remaining garlic, onion and paprika; cook, stirring, for 5 minutes. Add remaining wine, bay leaf, tomatoes, stock and reserved marinade.

4. Lock the lid in place and bring cooker up to full pressure over high heat. Reduce heat to medium-low, just to maintain even pressure, and cook for 20 minutes. Remove from heat and release pressure quickly. Discard bay leaf. If desired, simmer sauce, uncovered, to thicken. Stir in roasted pepper.

Swedish Meatballs

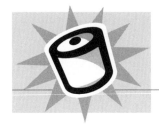

Serves 4

This classic combination is a hit with adults and kids alike. Serve the creamy sauce over lots of wide egg noodles.

1	slice whole wheat bread	1
1/2 cup	milk	125 mL
1 lb	extra-lean ground beef	500 g
8 oz	ground pork	250 g
1	egg	1
1	small onion, minced	1
1 tsp	dried dill	5 mL
1/2 tsp	salt	2 mL
1/4 cup	butter	50 mL
1/4 cup	all-purpose flour	50 mL
1	can (10 oz [284 mL]) beef broth diluted with equal amount of water	1
1/2 cup	whipping (35%) cream	125 mL
	Salt and freshly ground black pepper to taste	
	Cooked egg noodles	
2 tbsp	chopped fresh dill	25 mL

1. In a large bowl, soak bread in milk until absorbed. Using your hands, break up bread; mix in beef and pork. Stir in egg, minced onion, dried dill and salt. Form into 3/4-inch (2 cm) balls. Set aside.

2. In a pressure cooker, melt butter over medium-high heat; stir in flour until moistened. Gradually whisk in beef broth and water. Bring to a simmer. Carefully transfer meatballs to sauce.

3. Lock the lid in place and bring cooker up to full pressure over medium-high heat. Reduce heat to medium-low, just to maintain even pressure, and cook for 10 minutes. Remove from heat and release pressure quickly. Stir in cream and simmer until sauce is creamy and thick. Season to taste with salt and pepper. Serve over cooked egg noodles, sprinkled with fresh dill.

Lamb Curry with Lentils

Serves 4

This is a mild, Asian-style curry, flavored with coconut milk and thick-ened with red lentils. Serve it with lots of basmati rice, and a dish of steamed cauliflower or carrots on the side.

2 lbs	boneless lamb shoulder, fat removed, cut into 2-inch (5 cm) pieces	1 kg
1 tbsp	vegetable oil	15 mL
1 cup	chopped onions	250 mL
2	cloves garlic, crushed	2
2 tsp	minced ginger root	10 mL
2 tsp	curry powder	10 mL
1 tsp	salt	5 mL
1/4 tsp	ground cumin	1 mL
1/4 tsp	ground cloves	1 mL
1/4 tsp	ground cardamom	1 mL
1/4 tsp	freshly ground black pepper	1 mL
1/2 cup	diced tomatoes	125 mL
1/4 cup	dried red lentils	50 mL
1 cup	unsweetened coconut milk	250 mL
1/2 cup	beef stock	125 mL
1 tbsp	lemon juice	15 mL
1/4 cup	chopped cilantro or parsley	50 mL
4 cups	hot cooked basmati rice	1 L

1. In a pressure cooker, heat oil over medium-high heat. Add lamb in batches and cook until browned. Transfer to a bowl. Set aside.

2. Reduce heat to medium. Add onion, garlic, ginger, curry pow-der, salt, cumin, cloves, cardamom and pepper; sauté 2 minutes or until fragrant. Add tomatoes; cook for 1 minute. Stir in lentils, coconut milk, beef stock, lemon juice and lamb with any accumulated juices.

3. Lock the lid in place and bring cooker up to full pressure over high heat. Reduce heat to medium-low, just to maintain even pressure, and cook for 15 minutes. Remove from heat and release pressure quickly. Stir in cilantro. Serve over rice.

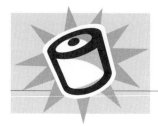

Saigon Braised Pork and Eggplant

Serves 6

The eggplant cooks down to form a thick, creamy sauce in this delicious Southeast Asian-style curry. Add another jalapeño pepper (or substitute hotter serrano or scotch bonnet chilies) if you like your food extra spicy, and serve over lots of fragrant jasmine or basmati rice.

TIP

If you're pressed for time, instead of simmering the sauce to thicken, whisk together 1 tbsp (15 mL) cornstarch with 1 tsp (5 mL) water; whisk into sauce. Cook, stirring, for about 3 minutes or until thickened.

2 lbs	country-style pork ribs or boneless pork steaks	1 kg
1 tbsp	vegetable oil *or* peanut oil	15 mL
4	cloves garlic, minced	4
1	onion, chopped	1
1	eggplant, cubed	1
1	jalapeño pepper, seeded and chopped	1
1	large carrot, cubed	1
1 cup	cubed waxy potatoes	250 mL
1 tbsp	granulated sugar	15 mL
1 tbsp	chopped ginger root	15 mL
1 tsp	curry powder	5 mL
1	star anise *or* 1/2 tsp (2 mL) anise seed	1
1 cup	water or chicken stock	250 mL
1/2 cup	chopped tomato (fresh or canned)	125 mL
1/4 cup	Thai *nuoc nam* or Vietnamese *nam pla* (fish sauce)	50 mL
1	bunch green onions, cut into 2-inch pieces	1
1/4 cup	chopped cilantro	50 mL

1. Cut pork ribs into 3-inch pieces. (If using steaks, cut into large chunks.) In a pressure cooker, heat oil over medium-high heat. Add pork in batches and cook for about 10 minutes until browned. Return pork to cooker. Add garlic and onion; cook, stirring, for 5 minutes. Stir in eggplant, jalapeño pepper, carrot, potatoes, sugar, ginger, curry powder, anise, water, tomato and fish sauce.

2. Lock the lid in place and bring cooker up to full pressure over high heat. Reduce heat to medium-low, just to maintain even pressure, and cook for 18 minutes. Remove from heat and release pressure quickly.

3. Simmer, uncovered, for 5 to 10 minutes until sauce is reduced and thickened. Discard star anise. Stir in green onions and cilantro. Serve immediately over rice.

Osso Buco

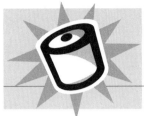

Serves 4

You can make this classic Italian dish with veal or lamb shanks. Ask the butcher to cut the shanks into 1 1/2-inch (4 cm) slices. Serve the osso buco with saffron-flavored Risotto (see recipe, page 142) or over creamy polenta flavored with Parmesan; add a robust red wine and you've got a rustic but elegant meal.

1/4 cup	all-purpose flour	50 mL
1/2 tsp	salt	2 mL
1/4 tsp	freshly ground black pepper	1 mL
4	slices veal or lamb shanks, about 1 1/2 inches (3 cm) thick	4
8	thin slices pancetta or smoked bacon	8
2 tbsp	olive oil	25 mL

SAUCE

2	stalks celery, minced	2
2	cloves garlic, minced	2
1	carrot, shredded	1
1	onion, minced	1
1	portobello mushroom, cut into strips (or substitute other flavorful varieties like shiitake, cepes, etc.)	1
1 tsp	dried thyme	5 mL
1	bay leaf	1
1 tsp	fresh or dried rosemary, minced	5 mL
1	bulb fennel, finely chopped *or* 1/2 tsp (2 mL) fennel seed	1
1 cup	dry red wine	250 mL
1 cup	tomato sauce	250 mL
	Salt and freshly ground black pepper to taste	

GREMOLATA

1/4 cup	chopped Italian parsley	50 mL
2	cloves garlic, minced	2
1/4 tsp	salt	1 mL
2 tsp	minced lemon zest	10 mL

1. In a plastic bag or bowl, combine flour with salt and pepper. Add veal and toss to coat. Wrap each piece in a slice of pancetta. Discard excess flour. In a pressure cooker, heat oil over medium-high heat. Add veal in batches and cook until browned. Transfer to a plate. Set aside.

2. Add celery, garlic, carrot, onion and mushroom to cooker; sauté for 2 minutes. Stir in thyme, bay leaf, rosemary, fennel, wine and tomato sauce, scraping up any browned bits from bottom of cooker. Nestle veal in sauce; pour in any accumulated juices.

3. Lock the lid in place and bring cooker up to full pressure over high heat. Reduce heat to medium-low, just to maintain even pressure, and cook for 15 minutes. Remove from heat and release pressure quickly. Transfer veal to a serving platter and tent with foil to keep warm. Discard bay leaf. If desired, simmer sauce, uncovered, to thicken. Season to taste with salt and pepper. Pour over veal.

4. GREMOLATA: In a small bowl, combine parsley, garlic, salt and lemon zest. Sprinkle on top of veal and serve with soft polenta.

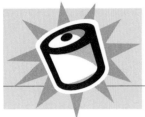

Round Steak Louisiana-Style

Serves 8

In Louisiana, this rich braised steak is called *grillades* and is often made with veal. The pressure cooker quickly tenderizes cuts like round steak making this a fast and inexpensive meal. Thicken the sauce after it's cooked with a light *roux* made of softened butter and flour, then serve steaks and sauce over grits or rice. Stir in fresh parsley and chopped green onions at the end for color and fresh flavor. For those who like their steak extra spicy, pass the Louisiana hot sauce.

4 lbs	inside or outside round steaks, about 1/2 inch (1 cm) thick, all visible fat removed	2 kg
8 oz	double-smoked bacon	250 g
	Vegetable oil	
3	cloves garlic, minced	3
1 1/2 cups	chopped green peppers	375 mL
1 cup	chopped onions	250 mL
3/4 cup	chopped celery	175 mL
2 cups	chopped tomatoes	500 mL
1 tsp	dried thyme	5 mL
1 cup	water	250 mL
1 cup	dry red wine	250 mL
2 tsp	salt	10 mL
2	bay leaves	2
1/2 tsp	freshly ground black pepper	2 mL
1/2 tsp	cayenne pepper	2 mL
2 tbsp	Worcestershire sauce	25 mL
1/4 cup	all-purpose flour	50 mL
1/4 cup	butter, softened	50 mL
1 cup	chopped green onions	250 mL
2 tbsp	chopped parsley	25 mL

1. Place meat between two sheets of waxed paper and, using a meat mallet, pound to 1/4-inch (5 mm) thickness. Cut into serving-sized pieces

2. In a pressure cooker over medium-high heat, cook bacon until crisp. Crumble and set aside. Add steaks in batches and brown on both sides, adding oil as necessary to prevent burning. Transfer to a bowl. Set aside.

3. Reduce heat to medium. Add garlic, green pepper, onions and celery; sauté for about 5 minutes or until softened. Add tomatoes and thyme; cook 3 minutes longer until tomatoes are starting to break down. Stir in water and wine. Return meat to cooker with accumulated juices, salt, bay leaves, pepper, cayenne and Worcestershire.

4. Lock the lid in place and bring cooker up to full pressure over high heat. Reduce heat to medium-low, just to maintain even pressure, and cook the meat for 15 minutes. Remove from heat and release pressure quickly. The meat should be fork tender. If not, return to full pressure and cook for 3 to 4 minutes longer. Remove from heat and release pressure quickly.

5. Transfer meat to a warmed serving platter and tent with foil to keep warm. Discard bay leaves. In a small bowl, mash flour with butter to form a smooth paste. Whisk into sauce and simmer, stirring, for about 5 minutes or until thickened. Stir in chopped green onions. Pour sauce over steak and garnish with reserved crumbled bacon and parsley.

Pork Loin with Calvados and Dried Fruit

Serves 4 to 6

The dried and fresh fruit in this recipe cooks down with the stock to create a thick, fruity gravy that's perfect with moist, juicy slices of roast pork. Make a mound of creamy mashed potatoes and some steamed green vegetables to round out this comforting meal.

2 tbsp	all-purpose flour	25 mL
1/2 tsp	salt	2 mL
1/4 tsp	freshly ground black pepper	1 mL
3 lb	boneless pork loin roast	1.5 kg
2 tbsp	olive oil	25 mL
1 1/2 cups	chicken stock	375 mL
1/4 cup	Calvados or brandy	50 mL
1	onion, chopped	1
1/2 cup	chopped rhubarb	125 mL
1/3 cup	chopped dried apricots	75 mL
1/3 cup	chopped pitted prunes	75 mL
1/3 cup	dried cranberries or currants	75 mL
1/2 tsp	dried thyme	2 mL
1/2 tsp	dried marjoram	2 mL
1 tsp	Worcestershire sauce	5 mL
	Salt and freshly ground black pepper to taste	

1. In a shallow dish, combine flour with salt and pepper. Roll pork loin in flour to coat all sides. Discard excess flour mixture.

2. In a pressure cooker, heat oil over medium-high heat. Add pork and brown on all sides. Stir in stock, Calvados, onion, rhubarb, apricots, prunes, cranberries, thyme, marjoram and Worcestershire.

3. Lock the lid in place and bring cooker up to full pressure over high heat. Reduce heat to medium-low, just to maintain even pressure, and cook for 40 minutes. Remove from heat and release pressure quickly. Check to make sure there is just a hint of pink remaining in pork. If not, return to full pressure and cook for 3 to 5 minutes longer, depending on doneness. Remove from heat and release pressure quickly.

4. Transfer pork to a warmed platter. Tent with foil and let rest for 10 minutes. Meanwhile, simmer the sauce, uncovered, to reduce slightly, stirring to break up the fruit. Season to taste with salt and pepper. Slice pork and serve drizzled with fruit sauce.

Slow-Roasted Beef Brisket with Chipotle Chili Rub

Serves 6 to 8

Chipotle chilies are jalapeños that have been roasted over a fire until they are deeply smoked. You can buy them in cans from Mexico in adobo sauce, or dried for reconstituting in warm water.

Look for chipotles in specialty or gourmet grocery stores (or in the produce sections of well-stocked supermarkets) or substitute 2 tsp (10 mL) Asian chili paste mixed with a few generous drops of liquid smoke.

This spicy beef pot roast is delicious served with creamy horseradish mashed potatoes, egg noodles, or chopped and folded into big flour tortillas.

2 tbsp	packed brown sugar	25 mL
1/2 tsp	ground cumin	2 mL
2	chipotle chilies in adobo sauce	2
3 tbsp	olive oil, divided	45 mL
2 tbsp	tomato paste	25 mL
1	beef brisket, about 3 lbs (1.5 kg), trimmed	1
1	large onion, sliced	1
3	cloves garlic, minced	3
1	can (14 oz [398 mL]) Mexican-style stewed tomatoes	1
1 tbsp	Worcestershire sauce	15 mL
1/2 tsp	salt	2 mL
1/4 tsp	freshly ground black pepper	1 mL

1. In a small bowl, mash sugar, cumin, chipotle chilies, 1 tbsp (15 mL) of the olive oil and tomato paste to form a smooth paste. In a zippered plastic bag or shallow dish, coat brisket with paste. Seal or cover and let stand at room temperature for 1 hour or refrigerate overnight.

2. Meanwhile, in a pressure cooker, heat remaining oil over medium-low heat. Add onions and cook, stirring, for about 10 minutes or until golden brown. Add garlic and cook 2 minutes longer. Stir in the tomatoes, Worcestershire, salt and pepper; simmer, uncovered, for 5 minutes. Place marinated brisket in sauce. Drizzle with any remaining marinade and spoon a little of the tomato sauce over top.

3. Lock the lid in place and bring cooker up to full pressure over high heat. Reduce the heat to medium-low, just to maintain even pressure, and cook for 1 hour. Remove from heat and allow pressure to drop naturally, for about 10 minutes, then release any remaining pressure quickly.

4. Transfer brisket to a warmed platter and tent with foil to keep warm. Bring sauce to boil; reduce heat and simmer for about 10 minutes or until reduced and thickened. Slice brisket thinly against the grain (or shred) and serve with the sauce.

Greek-Style Braised Lamb Shoulder

Serves 4

Start this recipe the night before to make sure the marinade infuses its flavors throughout the lamb. The perfect side dishes are boiled or roasted new potatoes and green vegetables like steamed beans or broccoli, lightly dressed with lemon and olive oil. Or try serving this tender lamb with steamed green beans and ROASTED GARLIC RISOTTO WITH ASIAGO, (see recipe, page 145).

3.5 to 4 lbs	lamb shoulder roast	1.75 to 2 kg
	Zest and juice of 1 large lemon (about 3 tbsp [45 mL] juice)	
3	cloves garlic, minced	3
1 tsp	dried oregano	5 mL
1/2 tsp	freshly ground black pepper	2 mL
1/4 cup	Dijon mustard	50 mL
1 cup	chopped onions	250 mL
3	bay leaves	3
2	cloves garlic, whole	2
1 tbsp	dried rosemary	15 mL
1 tsp	mustard seed	5 mL
1 cup	water	250 mL

1. Trim fat and sinew from the lamb and cut it into large, serving-size pieces. In a large bowl or zippered plastic bag, combine lemon zest and juice, minced garlic, oregano, pepper and mustard; add lamb and stir or toss to coat. Cover and refrigerate overnight.

2. In a pressure cooker, combine onions, bay leaves, garlic, rosemary and mustard seed. Add lamb and marinade. Pour in water.

3. Lock the lid in place and bring cooker up to full pressure over high heat. Reduce heat to medium-low, just to maintain pressure, and cook for 18 minutes. Remove from heat and release pressure quickly. The lamb should be very tender. If not, return to full pressure and cook for 2 to 3 minutes longer, depending on doneness. Remove from heat and release pressure quickly.

4. Remove meat from cooking juices and serve on a warm platter, surrounded with boiled or oven-roasted potatoes and vegetables.

Fish & Seafood

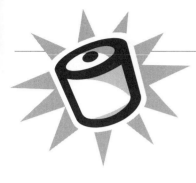

Steamed Salmon with Red Wine Glaze

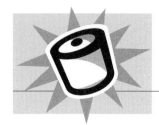

Serves 4

While there's not much time to save when cooking fish, the pressure cooker is nevertheless extremely fast and keeps the fish deliciously moist. Careful timing is critical for fish, however, to avoid overcooking. If you have a shallow sauté pan base for your cooker, use it when cooking fish to help cut down on the time it takes for the unit to reach full pressure.

4	pieces salmon fillet, skin on *or* 4 salmon steaks, about 2 lbs (1 kg)	4
1	small onion, sliced	1
1/2 cup	dry white wine	125 mL
1/2 cup	fish stock *or* clam juice *or* water	125 mL
2	sprigs thyme	2
2	sprigs parsley	2
	Salt to taste	

GLAZE

1 tbsp	brown sugar	15 mL
1/2 cup	orange juice	125 mL
1/2 cup	dry red wine	125 mL
1 tbsp	tomato paste	15 mL
1 tbsp	butter	15 mL

1. In a pressure cooker, combine onion, wine, stock, thyme and parsley; bring to a boil. Arrange fish in a single layer in cooker.

2. Lock the lid in place and bring cooker up to full pressure over high heat. Reduce heat to medium-low, just to maintain even pressure, and cook for 3 minutes. Remove from heat and release pressure quickly. The fish should flake easily with a fork. If not, return to full pressure and cook for 1 to 2 minutes longer. Remove from heat and release pressure quickly.

3. GLAZE: Meanwhile, in a small saucepan, combine sugar, orange juice, wine and tomato paste. Bring to boil over high heat; cook until reduced to 1/3 cup (75 mL). Whisk in butter and keep warm.

4. Transfer salmon to individual serving plates. Season with salt to taste. Spoon some of the red wine glaze over each serving.

Halibut Steaks with Peppers

Serves 4

Try making this colorful dish in the late summer, when there are lots of pretty peppers in the market. Add a couple of banana peppers for extra spice.

TIP

If halibut is unavailable, use another firm-fleshed fish, such as salmon or swordfish.

1/4 cup	extra virgin olive oil	50 mL
1	red bell pepper, sliced	1
1	yellow bell pepper, sliced	1
1 cup	zucchini, cut into matchsticks	250 mL
1 tsp	minced garlic	5 mL
1/2 cup	sliced shallots or leeks	125 mL
1 tbsp	minced thyme	15 mL
1 tbsp	minced rosemary	15 mL
4	halibut steaks, 3/4 inch (3 cm) thick, about 1 1/2 lbs (750 g) total	4
1 cup	white wine	250 mL
1/2 tsp	salt	2 mL
1/4 tsp	freshly ground black pepper	1 mL
	Sprigs of thyme or rosemary	

1. In a pressure cooker, heat oil over high heat. Add red and yellow peppers, zucchini, garlic and shallots; sauté for about 10 minutes or until vegetables start to brown. Stir in thyme and rosemary.

2. Place fish in a single layer on the vegetables and pour in wine. Sprinkle with salt and pepper.

3. Lock the lid in place and bring cooker up to full pressure over high heat. Reduce heat to medium-low, just to maintain even pressure, and cook for 3 to 4 minutes. Remove from heat and release pressure quickly. The fish should flake easily with a fork. If not, return to full pressure and cook for 1 to 2 minutes longer. Remove from heat and release pressure quickly.

4. Serve fish in shallow bowls with rice, topped with the mixed vegetables and a drizzle of the braising liquid. Garnish with sprigs of thyme or rosemary.

Braised Sea Bass
Provençal

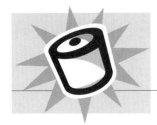

Serves 4

The browning of both the fish and the vegetables adds an extra layer of flavor to the final dish.

4	pieces sea bass fillet, 1 1/2 inches (3 cm) thick, about 1 1/2 lbs (750 g)	4
1 tbsp	all-purpose flour	15 mL
3 tbsp	extra virgin olive oil	45 mL
2	leeks, white parts only, halved and sliced	2
3	cloves garlic, coarsely chopped	3
2	carrots, thinly sliced	2
1	bulb fennel, white part only, trimmed and slivered	1
1 cup	small white mushrooms, halved	250 mL
Half	red or yellow bell pepper, diced	Half
1	large plum tomato, seeded and chopped	1
1/2 tsp	dried thyme	2 mL
1/2 tsp	dried oregano	2 mL
1/2 tsp	salt	2 mL
1/2 tsp	freshly ground black pepper	2 mL
1/4 cup	chicken stock	50 mL
1/4 cup	white wine	50 mL
2 tbsp	chopped Italian parsley	25 mL
1 to 2 tsp	cornstarch dissolved in 1 tsp (5 mL) water (optional)	5 to 10 mL

1. Remove skin from sea bass, if desired. Dust each fillet on one side with flour. In a pressure cooker, heat oil over high heat until almost smoking. In batches, cook fish, floured-side down, for 1 minute or just until golden brown. Transfer to a plate. Set aside.

2. Reduce heat to medium. Add leeks, garlic, carrot, fennel and mushrooms; cook, stirring, for 5 minutes or until beginning to brown and caramelize. Add red pepper and sauté 1 minute longer. Stir in tomato, thyme, oregano, salt and pepper; cook for 30 seconds. Place fish, browned-side up, on top of vegetables; pour in chicken stock and wine.

3. Lock the lid in place and bring cooker up to full pressure over high heat. Reduce heat to medium-low, just to maintain even pressure, and cook for 3 to 4 minutes, depending on thickness of fish. Remove from heat and release pressure quickly. The fish should flake easily with a fork. If not, return to full pressure and cook for 1 to 2 minutes longer. Remove from heat and release pressure quickly.

4. Transfer fish to a platter and tent with foil to keep warm. If desired, whisk cornstarch mixture into sauce. Bring to a boil; reduce heat and simmer, stirring, until slightly thickened. Spoon sauce over each serving of fish and vegetables. Sprinkle with chopped parsley.

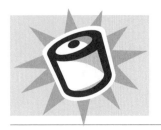

Spanish Cod and Mussel Stew with Tomatoes and Green Olives

Serves 4

The pressure cooker instantly infuses and mingles the flavors of this Mediterranean-inspired fish stew. The mixture is hot enough to perfectly steam the mussels at the end without any additional cooking. Serve the stew over polenta or with plenty of French bread.

TIP

Before cooking, inspect mussels and discard any that do not fully close when tapped. After cooking, discard any mussels that have not opened.

1/4 cup	extra virgin olive oil	50 mL
1	onion, finely chopped	1
2	cloves garlic, minced	1
1 tsp	sweet Spanish paprika	5 mL
1/4 tsp	cayenne pepper	1 mL
1/4 tsp	crushed saffron threads	1 mL
1/2 cup	dry white wine	125 mL
1	can (14 oz [398 mL]) plum tomatoes, chopped	1
2 oz	prosciutto, cut into slivers	50 g
1/2 cup	sliced green olives	125 mL
2 lbs	firm white cod (*or* monkfish *or* sea bass), cut into 2-inch (5 cm) chunks	1 kg
2 lbs	mussels, scrubbed and debearded	1 kg
1/4 tsp	salt	1 mL
1/4 tsp	freshly ground black pepper	1 mL

1. In a pressure cooker, heat oil over medium heat. Add onion and sauté until soft. Stir in garlic, paprika and cayenne; sauté for 1 minute. Add saffron, wine, tomatoes, prosciutto and green olives. Stir in the fish.

2. Lock the lid in place and bring cooker up to full pressure over high heat. Reduce heat to low, just to maintain even pressure, and cook for 3 minutes. Remove from heat and release pressure quickly.

3. Add mussels to cooker; cover, but don't lock the lid in place. Bring to a boil, then set aside, covered, for 5 minutes until mussels open. Stir in salt and pepper.

4. Serve stew in deep soup bowls over polenta, or with lots of crusty bread for sopping up the juices.

East-West Curried Seafood Stew

Serves 4 to 6

This is a bouillabaisse with Southeast Asian overtones. It's rich and creamy – the perfect dish for those times when you feel like something a little exotic. Try serving it in shallow bowls over mounds of fragrant basmati or jasmine rice.

2	cloves garlic, minced	2
1	apple, peeled and chopped	1
1	banana, peeled and sliced	1
1/2 cup	raisins	125 mL
1/4 cup	curry powder	50 mL
2 tbsp	brown sugar	25 mL
1/4 tsp	ground cumin	1 mL
1/4 tsp	crushed saffron threads	1 mL
2 cups	unsweetened coconut milk	500 mL
2 cups	chicken stock	500 mL
2 tbsp	lemon or lime juice	25 mL
1 tsp	Worcestershire sauce	5 mL
3/4 cup	whipping (35%) cream	175 mL
12	large mussels, scrubbed and debearded	12
16	large prawns, peeled and deveined	16
16	sea scallops	16
12 oz	snapper (*or* halibut *or* other firm white fish), cubed	375 g
1/2 cup	cooked chickpeas (see table, page 17)	125 mL
1/2 cup	diced red bell pepper	125 mL
1/4 cup	chopped cilantro	50 mL

1. In a pressure cooker, combine garlic, apple, banana, raisins, curry powder, brown sugar, cumin, saffron, coconut milk, stock, lemon juice and Worcestershire.

2. Lock the lid in place and bring cooker up to full pressure over high heat. Reduce heat to medium-low, just to maintain even pressure, and cook for 10 minutes. Remove from heat and release pressure quickly.

3. Using an immersion blender or food processor, purée the soup. (If using a food processor, allow soup to cool slightly, then process in batches.) Stir in cream. Add mussels, prawns, scallops, fish, chickpeas and red peppers.

4. Lock the lid in place and bring cooker up to full pressure over medium-high heat. Reduce heat to medium-low, just to maintain even pressure, and cook for 2 minutes. Remove from heat and release pressure quickly.

5. Divide fish and seafood between 4 deep soup bowls. Ladle soup over top and sprinkle each serving with cilantro.

Cajun Seafood Gumbo

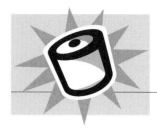

Serves 6 to 8

This is truly a meal-in-a-bowl. Boil some rice to serve in the middle of deep serving bowls, and ladle the soup/stew over top. If you don't live in an area where fresh crab is available, substitute frozen or canned crab meat. If your oysters arrive shucked in a jar, add the oyster liquor to the stew.

1/2 cup	vegetable oil, divided	125 mL
1 cup	chopped onions	250 mL
3/4 cup	chopped celery	175 mL
1 cup	chopped red bell pepper	250 mL
2 tbsp	minced garlic	25 mL
1/2 cup	all-purpose flour	125 mL
8 oz	smoked andouille sausages, sliced (or substitute any spicy smoked sausage)	250 g
6 cups	fish stock (see recipe, page 176)	1.5 L
2 tbsp	dried thyme	25 mL
1/2 tsp	freshly ground black pepper	2 mL
1 lb	large shrimp, peeled and deveined	500 g
1 lb	lump crabmeat or crawfish meat	500 g
24	oysters, shucked	24
	Salt and cayenne pepper to taste	
1/2 cup	chopped green onions	125 mL
1/4 cup	chopped parsley	50 mL
6 to 8 cups	hot cooked rice	1.5 to 2 L

1. In a pressure cooker, heat 2 tbsp (25 mL) of the oil over medium heat. Stir in onions, red pepper, celery and garlic; sauté for 5 minutes until vegetables are beginning to brown. Stir in sausage, thyme, black pepper and fish stock.

2. Lock the lid in place and bring cooker up to full pressure over high heat. Reduce heat to medium-low, just to maintain even pressure, and cook for 10 minutes. Remove from heat and release pressure quickly.

3. In a saucepan, heat remaining oil over medium-low heat. Sprinkle in flour and cook, stirring constantly, until the *roux* turns the color of peanut butter, about 12 minutes. (Be careful – this gets very hot and burns easily.) Remove from heat and let cool slightly.

4. Whisk some of the broth into the *roux* and pour mixture into cooker; cook, stirring, until nicely thickened. Add shrimp, crabmeat and oysters.

5. Lock the lid in place and bring cooker up to full pressure over medium-high heat. Cook for 1 minute. Remove from heat and release pressure quickly.

6. Season to taste with salt and cayenne pepper. Stir in green onions and parsley. Heat through before serving.

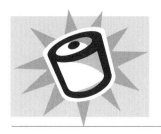

Steamed Rock Cod with Fermented Black Beans and Miso

Serves 4

This is a light and flavorful way to serve fish. Make some fragrant Thai rice and stir-fried bok choy with sesame seeds to serve alongside.

7- OR 8-INCH (18 OR 20 CM) GLASS PIE PLATE (USE SMALLER SIZE IF NECESSARY TO FIT INSIDE PRESSURE COOKER)

RACK OR TRIVET TO FIT BOTTOM OF PRESSURE COOKER

2 lbs	rock cod or red snapper fillets	1 kg
1 tsp	salt	5 mL
1 tbsp	red miso paste	15 mL
1 tbsp	rice wine	15 mL
2 tsp	fermented black beans	10 mL
2 tsp	sesame oil	10 mL
1 tsp	dark soy sauce	5 mL
1/2 tsp	Asian chili paste	2 mL
1	2-inch (5 cm) piece ginger root, cut into matchsticks	1
2	cloves garlic, minced	2
4	green onions, halved lengthwise and cut into 2-inch (5 cm) pieces	4

1. In a shallow glass dish, rub fish on all sides with salt. In a bowl combine miso, rice wine, black beans, sesame oil, soy sauce and chili paste. Rub mixture over both sides of fillets. Let stand for 10 minutes.

2. Sprinkle bottom of pie plate with half of the ginger, half of the garlic and half of the green onions; arrange fish fillets over top. Drizzle with any remaining sauce and sprinkle with remaining ginger, garlic and green onions. Set rack in bottom of cooker. Pour in enough water to fill just below top of rack. Place pie plate on rack.

3. Lock the lid in place and bring cooker up to full pressure over high heat. Reduce heat to medium-low, just to maintain even pressure, and cook for 3 minutes. Remove from heat and release pressure quickly. Serve immediately.

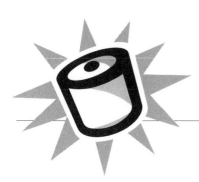

Vegetarian and Salads

Warm Lemon Lentil Salad

Serves 4 to 6

Use the regular brown or green lentils in this dish or the smaller French green lentils if you can find them.

Lentil salad is a traditional French first course but also makes a nice base for grilled fish or lamb chops.

TIP

In place of the fresh herb bundle, use a tea ball containing 1 tsp (5 mL) dried thyme, 1 tsp (5 mL) dried rosemary and a bay leaf. Remove from cooker at the end of Step 2.

1	sprig thyme	1
1	sprig rosemary	1
1	bay leaf	1
1 cup	brown or green lentils	250 mL
2	cloves garlic, peeled	2
1	carrot, quartered	1
3 cups	water	750 mL
1 tbsp	vegetable oil	15 mL

DRESSING

	Zest of 1 lemon, minced	
	Juice of 1 lemon (about 3 tbsp [45 mL] juice)	
2 tsp	chopped thyme (or 1 tsp [5 mL] dried)	10 mL
1	clove garlic, minced	1
1 tsp	salt	5 mL
1 tbsp	Dijon mustard	15 mL
1/4 cup	extra virgin olive oil	50 mL
	Freshly ground black pepper	
4	plum tomatoes, seeded and chopped	4
3	green onions, chopped	3
1/4 cup	chopped parsley	50 mL
	Mixed greens	

1. Using kitchen string, tie thyme, rosemary and bay leaf into a bundle. In a pressure cooker, combine herb bundle, lentils, garlic, carrot, water and oil.

2. Lock the lid in place and bring cooker up to full pressure over high heat. Reduce heat to medium-low, just to maintain even pressure, and cook for 8 minutes. Remove from heat and allow pressure to drop naturally. Drain well. Discard herb bundle, carrot and garlic. Transfer lentils to a bowl.

3. DRESSING: In a bowl whisk together lemon zest, lemon juice, thyme, garlic, salt and mustard. Slowly whisk in olive oil to emulsify. Season with pepper to taste.

4. Pour dressing over the lentils and toss to coat. Stir in tomatoes, green onions and parsley. Serve salad warm over mixed greens or as a base for grilled meat or fish.

Chickpea Salad with Roasted Onions and Bell Peppers

Serves 4

This flavorful and healthy salad is ideal for taking to a picnic or to carry on a hike. The salad is delicious on the day you make it, but just as good the next day. You'll be amazed how toothsome and delicious chickpeas can be when cooked from scratch in the pressure cooker.

1 cup	dried chickpeas	250 mL
4 cups	water	1 L
1	red bell pepper	1
2 tsp	olive oil	10 mL
1	large onion	1
1	head garlic	1
2	plum tomatoes, seeded and chopped	2
1 tbsp	chopped thyme (or 1 tsp [5 mL] dried)	15 mL
1 tbsp	chopped sage leaves (or 1 tsp [5 mL] dried)	15 mL
1 tsp	sea salt	5 mL
1/2 tsp	freshly ground black pepper	2 mL
1/2 tsp	cayenne pepper	2 mL
1/4 cup	extra virgin olive oil	50 mL
3 tbsp	lemon juice	45 mL
1/4 cup	minced Italian parsley	50 mL

1. Soak chickpeas overnight in water to cover or use the quick pressure-soak method, page 130. Drain.

2. In a pressure cooker, combine chickpeas and water. Lock the lid in place and bring cooker up to full pressure over high heat. Reduce heat to medium-low, just to maintain even pressure, and cook for 15 minutes. Remove from heat and allow pressure to drop naturally. Drain. Transfer to a large bowl.

3. Meanwhile, on the barbecue or under the broiler, char the red pepper. Place in a bag to cool. Peel off skin, remove seeds and chop. Add to chickpeas in bowl. Wrap onion and garlic, unpeeled, in a piece of foil and drizzle with olive oil. Roast in a preheated 400° F (200° C) oven for 45 minutes or until very soft. Peel onion and cut into slivers; add to chickpeas in bowl. Squeeze garlic out of skins into the bowl.

4. Add tomatoes, thyme, sage, salt, pepper, cayenne, olive oil and lemon juice; toss to coat. Cool to room temperature and let stand for 1 hour to allow flavors to meld. Just before serving, stir in parsley.

Barley Risotto Primavera

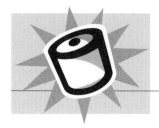

Serves 6

This dish is just like the famous Italian specialty, but made with whole barley for a unique prairie twist.

TIP

To save preparation time, mince onion, garlic, zucchini, carrot and celery in a food processor.

2 tbsp	olive oil	25 mL
1 cup	pearl or pot barley	250 mL
1	small onion, minced	1
1	clove garlic, minced	1
1/2 cup	finely chopped zucchini	125 mL
1/4 cup	minced carrot	50 mL
1/4 cup	minced celery	50 mL
2 1/2 cups	vegetable stock *or* water	625 mL
1 tsp	tamari soy sauce	5 mL
1/4 cup	freshly grated Parmesan cheese	50 mL
1/8 tsp	freshly ground black pepper	0.5 mL

1. In a pressure cooker, heat oil over medium heat. Add barley and sauté for 1 minute or until toasted. Add onion, garlic, zucchini, carrot and celery; sauté for 1 minute longer or until vegetables begin to soften. Stir in the stock and soy sauce.

2. Lock the lid in place and bring cooker up to full pressure over high heat. Reduce heat to medium-low, just to maintain even pressure, and cook for 18 minutes. Remove from heat and allow pressure to drop naturally.

3. Fluff risotto with a spoon. Stir in Parmesan cheese and pepper. Serve immediately.

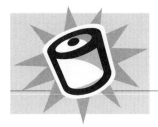

Chestnuts with Red Cabbage and Apples

Serves 4 to 6

This dish makes a nice accompaniment to grilled sausages, baked ham or roast goose, and is a nice holiday alternative to the usual Brussels sprouts. Despite their rich flavor, chestnuts are actually low in fat.

TIP

The pressure cooker makes peeling chestnuts fast and easy. Cut an X in the base of each nut and place in the cooker; cover nuts with plenty of water, lock lid in place, and cook at high pressure for 6 minutes. You'll find it's easy to peel off the shells and the brown, papery skin (which is bitter).

You can also use your pressure cooker to speed-soak the smoky-flavored dried chestnuts sold in Italian and Asian markets throughout the year. Allow 2 minutes of cooking under pressure and 10 minutes of natural pressure release to rehydrate the dried chestnuts.

2 tbsp	butter	25 mL
1	onion, chopped	1
1 lb	shredded red cabbage	500 g
2	green apples, peeled and cut into wedges	2
1 cup	peeled fresh chestnuts *or* rehydrated dried chestnuts (see Tip, at left)	250 mL
1 tsp	salt	5 mL
1/2 cup	dry white wine	125 mL
1/2 cup	water *or* chicken stock	125 mL
1/4 tsp	freshly ground black pepper	1 mL

1. In a pressure cooker, melt butter over medium heat. Add onions and sauté for 5 minutes or until softened. Add cabbage, stirring to coat with butter. Add apples, chestnuts, salt, wine and water.

2. Lock the lid in place and bring cooker up to full pressure over high heat. Reduce heat to medium-low, just to maintain even pressure, and cook for 10 minutes. Remove from heat and release pressure quickly.

3. Simmer, uncovered, until liquid is reduced. Stir in pepper and serve immediately.

Chickpea and Mixed Vegetable Stew

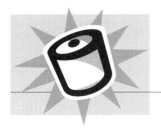

Serves 8

This substantial stew provides a gardenful of healthy vegetables in one pot. Here's proof positive that vegetarian food can be hearty enough for the coldest winter day.

1 cup	dried chickpeas	250 mL
4 cups	water	1 L
2 tbsp	olive oil	25 mL
3	cloves garlic, minced	3
2	stalks celery, chopped	2
1	onion, chopped	1
2	large potatoes, peeled and chopped	2
1	red bell pepper, chopped	1
1	large carrot, chopped	1
1/2 cup	small red lentils	125 mL
2 cups	vegetable stock	500 mL
1/2 cup	dry white wine	125 mL
3 tbsp	chopped basil *or* basil pesto	45 mL
1 tbsp	chopped rosemary	15 mL
	Salt and freshly ground black pepper to taste	
2 cups	polenta, cooked (see recipe, facing page)	500 mL
	Extra virgin olive oil for drizzling	
1/2 cup	freshly grated Parmesan cheese	125 mL

1. Soak chickpeas overnight in water to cover or use the quick pressure-soak method, page 130. Drain.

2. In a pressure cooker, combine chickpeas and water. Lock the lid in place and bring cooker up to full pressure over high heat. Reduce heat to medium-low, just to maintain even pressure, and cook for 14 minutes. Remove from heat and allow pressure drop naturally. Drain. Set aside.

3. Wipe cooker clean. Add oil and heat over medium heat. Add garlic, celery and onion; sauté until onion is soft. Add potatoes, red pepper and carrot; toss to coat with oil. Add chickpeas, lentils, stock and wine.

4. Lock the lid in place and bring cooker up to full pressure over high heat. Reduce heat to medium-low, just to maintain even pressure, and cook for 5 minutes. Remove from heat and allow pressure to drop naturally.

5. Stir in basil and rosemary. Heat, uncovered, over low heat for 5 minutes; season to taste with salt and pepper. Serve stew in deep bowls over a mound of soft polenta, drizzled with extra virgin olive oil and sprinkled with Parmesan.

POLENTA

8 cups	water	2 L
2 cups	coarsely ground corn meal	500 mL
4 tbsp	butter	50 mL
1/2 cup	finely grated Parmesan cheese	125 mL

1. In large heavy-bottomed saucepan, bring water to a boil; reduce heat to low. Add cornmeal in a slow, thin stream, whisking constantly. With a wooden spoon, stir every minute or so until the mixture pulls away from the side of the pan in one mass. Depending on coarseness of cornmeal, this will take from 5 to 20 minutes. Stir in butter and cheese.

Vegetable Couscous

Serves 4

Couscous is one of those wonderful accompaniments that add interest to everyday meals without a lot of fuss. This is an almost-instant vegetarian meal in a pot, featuring plenty of healthy vegetables and exotic Moroccan flavors.

1 cup	dried chickpeas	250 mL
4 cups	cold water	1 L
2 tbsp	olive oil	25 mL
1	onion, chopped	1
1	clove garlic, minced	1
1	red or yellow bell pepper, chopped	1
2 tsp	ground cumin	10 mL
1 tsp	Hungarian paprika	5 mL
1/2 tsp	salt	2 mL
1/4 tsp	freshly ground black pepper	1 mL
1/4 tsp	ground cinnamon	1 mL
1/8 tsp	cayenne pepper	0.5 mL
1/4 cup	currants or raisins	50 mL
2 cups	vegetable stock	500 mL
1 1/2 cups	couscous	325 mL
1	small zucchini, diced	1
1 cup	frozen green peas, thawed	250 mL
3 tbsp	chopped fresh cilantro	45 mL

1. Soak chickpeas overnight in water to cover or use the quick pressure-soak method, page 130. Drain.

2. In a pressure cooker, combine chickpeas with water. Lock the lid in place and bring cooker up to full pressure over high heat. Reduce heat to medium-low, just to maintain even pressure, and cook for 14 minutes. Remove from heat and allow pressure drop naturally. Drain. Set aside.

3. Wipe cooker clean. Add oil and heat over medium heat. Add onions, garlic and red pepper; sauté for 5 minutes or until softened. Stir in cumin, paprika, salt, pepper, cinnamon and cayenne; cook for 2 minutes longer. Stir in chickpeas and raisins. Pour in stock.

4. Lock the lid in place and bring cooker up to full pressure over high heat. Reduce heat to medium-low, just to maintain even pressure, and cook for 4 minutes. Remove from heat and release pressure quickly.

5. Stir in couscous, zucchini and peas. Let stand, covered, for 10 minutes. Fluff with a fork and stir in the cilantro.

Biryani

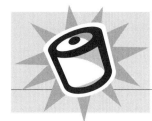

*Serves 2 as a main dish
or 4 as a side dish*

You can add almost any vegetable or meat to this wonderful Indian rice dish. It makes the perfect accompaniment to tandoori chicken or grilled lamb. And while this version is vegetarian, feel free to experiment by adding cooked meats to make it into a non-vegetarian main dish. Stir in cooked leftover chicken, beef or lamb after releasing pressure, then heat through before serving.

TIP

Garam masala is an Indian spice mixture that you can find in the Asian section of most large supermarkets.

2 tbsp	vegetable oil	25 mL
2 tsp	salt	10 mL
2 tsp	sweet Spanish or Hungarian paprika	10 mL
2 tsp	turmeric	10 mL
2 tsp	garam masala	10 mL
1/2 tsp	cayenne pepper	2 mL
1	onion, halved and sliced	1
1/2 cup	small mushrooms, halved	125 mL
Half	green pepper, diced	Half
1 cup	basmati rice	250 mL
1/2 cup	small florets cauliflower	125 mL
1/2 cup	diced carrots	125 mL
1/4 cup	chopped dried apricots or raisins	50 mL
2 cups	water *or* vegetable stock	500 mL
1/2 cup	frozen peas, thawed	125 mL

1. In a pressure cooker, heat oil over low heat. Add salt, paprika, turmeric, garam masala and cayenne; cook, stirring, for 1 minute.

2. Increase heat to medium. Add onion, mushrooms and green pepper; sauté for 2 to 3 minutes or until the mushrooms begin to give up their liquid. Stir in rice, cauliflower, carrots and raisins. Pour in water.

3. Lock the lid in place and bring cooker up to full pressure over high heat. Reduce heat to medium-low, just to maintain even pressure, and cook for 7 minutes. Remove from heat and allow pressure to drop naturally for 2 minutes; release remaining pressure quickly.

4. Stir in the peas. Replace cover on cooker (but do not lock) and let steam for 5 minutes. Fluff with a fork.

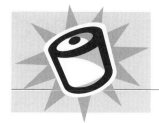

Caribbean Red Beans and Barley

Serves 6 to 8

Here's a flavorful combination of Canadian beans and barley, with a burst of Island heat. It's the perfect side dish for JAMAICAN CHICKEN FRICASEE (see recipe, page 66).

TIP

Use pearl or hulled barley; in a pressure cooker, pearl barley needs about 7 minutes to cook, while hulled barley takes twice as long, about 15 minutes.

1 cup	dried red kidney beans	250 mL
2	cloves garlic, minced	2
2	stalks celery, chopped	2
1	small onion, chopped	1
4 cups	water	1 L
1 1/2 cups	pearl or hulled barley (see Tip, at left)	375 mL
1	whole scotch bonnet pepper *or* 2 whole jalapeño peppers	1
2 tsp	dried thyme	10 mL
2 cups	unsweetened coconut milk	500 mL
3	green onions, minced	3
1 tbsp	butter	15 mL
	Salt and white pepper to taste	

1. Soak beans overnight in water to cover or use the quick pressure-soak method, page 130. Drain.

2. In a pressure cooker, combine beans, garlic, celery, onion and water. Lock the lid in place and bring cooker up to full pressure over high heat. Reduce heat to medium-low, just to maintain even pressure, and cook for 10 minutes. Remove from heat and allow pressure to drop naturally.

3. Stir in barley, scotch bonnet pepper, thyme and coconut milk. Lock the lid in place and bring cooker up to full pressure over high heat. Reduce heat to medium-low, just to maintain even pressure, and cook 7 minutes for pearl barley, 15 minutes for hulled barley. Remove from heat and allow pressure to drop naturally.

4. Discard scotch bonnet pepper. Stir in green onions and butter. Season to taste with salt and white pepper. Serve immediately.

Creamy Lentils and Cheddar

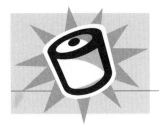

Serves 4

This vegetarian dish is simple and homey – your high-fiber alternative to mac and cheese. Try it as a side dish with sliced grilled bratwurst, European frankfurters or ham.

2	cloves garlic, minced	2
1 cup	brown or green lentils	250 mL
1 cup	chopped onions	250 mL
1	carrot, grated	1
1	yellow or red bell pepper, minced	1
1	bay leaf	1
1/2 tsp	dried thyme	2 mL
1	can (14 oz [398 mL]) tomatoes, puréed	1
1 cup	water	250 mL
1/2 cup	whipping (35%) cream	125 mL
1 cup	grated old Cheddar cheese	250 mL

1. In a pressure cooker, combine garlic, lentils, onions, carrot, red pepper, bay leaf, thyme, tomatoes and water. Make sure cooker is no more than half full.

2. Lock the lid in place and bring cooker up to full pressure over high heat. Reduce heat to medium-low, just to maintain even pressure, and cook for 10 minutes. Remove from heat and allow pressure to drop naturally. The lentils should be tender. If not, return to full pressure and cook for 2 to 4 minutes longer. Remove from heat and allow pressure to drop naturally.

3. Discard bay leaf. Stir in cream and bring to a boil. Reduce heat and simmer until the sauce is thickened. Remove from heat and add cheese; stir gently until cheese is melted and combined.

Boston 'Baked' Beans

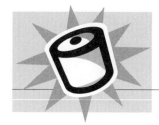

Serves 6

While this pressure-cooker version of classic baked beans is vegetarian, feel free to add about 8 oz (125 mL) sautéed chopped bacon or salt pork for a richer, more traditional flavor.

3 cups	dried white navy beans *or* Great Northern beans	500 mL
6 1/2 cups	water	1.625 L
2 tbsp	olive oil	25 mL
1/4 cup	packed brown sugar	50 mL
1/4 cup	molasses	50 mL
2 tbsp	Dijon mustard	25 mL
1 cup	chopped onions	250 mL
2	cloves garlic, minced	2
1 cup	tomato sauce	250 mL
1/4 tsp	freshly ground black pepper	1 mL
1 to 2 tsp	salt (or to taste)	5 to 10 mL

1. Soak beans overnight in water to cover or use the quick pressure-soak method, page 130. Drain.

2. In a pressure cooker, combine beans with 6 cups (1.5 L) of the water. Lock the lid in place and bring cooker up to full pressure over high heat. Reduce heat to medium-low, just to maintain even pressure, and cook 6 minutes for navy beans or 10 minutes for Great Northern. Remove from heat and allow pressure to drop naturally. Drain.

3. Whisk remaining water into cooker, together with the garlic, onion, brown sugar, pepper, tomato sauce, oil, molasses and mustard. Stir in beans.

4. Lock the lid in place and bring cooker up to full pressure over high heat. Reduce heat to medium-low, just to maintain even pressure, and cook for 2 minutes. Remove from heat and allow pressure to drop naturally. The beans should be tender. If not, add a little water (if necessary) and lock the lid in place. Return to full pressure and cook for 2 to 3 minutes longer. Remove from heat and allow pressure to drop naturally.

5. Drain off any excess liquid or let beans sit, covered, for 30 minutes until more of the liquid is absorbed. Season to taste with salt.

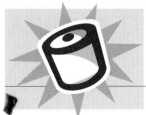

Vegetarian Barley, Lentil and Black Bean Chili

Serves 6

Here's a great alternative to traditional meat-based chili. The beans, lentils and grains combine to form a complete protein – plus a chewy, meaty texture that will satisfy any carnivore.

TIP

Choose a jalapeño pepper for a modest amount of heat. For extra fire, use a scotch bonnet pepper.

2 tbsp	vegetable oil	25 mL
3	cloves garlic, minced	3
1	large Spanish onion, chopped	1
1	jalapeño, scotch bonnet or serrano chili, seeded and minced	1
1 cup	brown or green lentils	250 mL
1 cup	cooked black beans (see page 17 for cooking times)	250 mL
1 cup	pearl barley	250 mL
3 tbsp	chili powder	45 mL
1 tbsp	sweet Hungarian paprika	15 mL
1 tsp	dried oregano	5 mL
1 tsp	ground cumin	5 mL
6 cups	vegetable stock	1.5 L
1	chipotle pepper in adobo sauce, chopped	1
1	can (28 oz [796 mL]) plum tomatoes, crushed	1
	Salt and freshly ground black pepper	

1. In a pressure cooker, heat oil over medium heat. Add garlic and onion; sauté until tender. Add chili pepper and sauté for 1 minute. Stir in lentils, black beans, barley, chili powder, paprika, oregano, cumin, stock, chipotle pepper and tomatoes.

2. Lock the lid in place and bring cooker up to full pressure over high heat. Reduce heat to medium-low, just to maintain even pressure, and cook for 10 minutes. Remove from heat and allow pressure to drop naturally for 10 minutes. Release any remaining pressure quickly. The barley and lentils should be tender. If not, return to full pressure for 2 to 3 minutes longer. Remove from heat and allow pressure to drop naturally.

3. Simmer, uncovered, until thickened. Season to taste with salt and pepper.

Curried Lentils with Spinach

Serves 4

With a pressure cooker, this classic Indian dish is ready in a fraction of the time normally required to prepare it. Serve as a side dish with an Indian meal, as a healthy accompaniment to lamb or pork, or simply over a pile of Basmati rice.

2 tbsp	vegetable oil	25 mL
2	dried hot peppers, crushed	2
1/2 tsp	cumin seeds	2 mL
1/2 tsp	ground coriander	2 mL
1/2 tsp	mustard seed or dried mustard	2 mL
2	cloves garlic, minced	2
1	onion, minced	1
1	large tomato, seeded and chopped	1
1 tbsp	minced ginger root	15 mL
1 cup	brown or green lentils	250 mL
1/2 tsp	salt	2 mL
3 1/2 cups	water	875 mL
2 tbsp	lemon juice	25 mL
2 cups	fresh spinach, washed thoroughly and finely chopped (or 1 package frozen chopped spinach, thawed and squeezed dry)	500 mL
	Coriander chutney or mango chutney as a condiment	

1. In a pressure cooker, heat oil over medium heat. Add hot peppers, cumin seed, mustard seed and coriander; sauté for about 20 seconds or until fragrant. Add onion, garlic, tomato and ginger; sauté for 3 minutes or until vegetables are soft and tomato begins to break down. Stir in lentils, salt, water, lemon juice and spinach.

2. Lock the lid in place and bring cooker up to full pressure over high heat. Reduce heat to medium-low, just to maintain even pressure, and cook for 12 minutes. Remove from heat and allow pressure to drop naturally.

3. Simmer, uncovered, to reduce liquid if necessary. Serve over basmati rice with a dollop of coriander or mango chutney on the side.

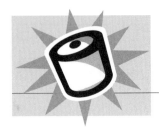

Spanish Potatoes and Chickpeas

Serves 4 as a main course or 8 to 10 for tapas

With its rich, garlicky saffron sauce, this dish is the ultimate vegetarian comfort food. Serve it in little bowls with crusty bread for a hot tapas starter, as an everyday main course, or as an exotic side dish with fried fish. For a more substantial (non-vegetarian) version, fry 1/2 cup (125 mL) chopped chorizo sausage or prosciutto ham with the onions and potatoes.

1 cup	dried chickpeas	250 mL
1/4 cup	olive oil	50 mL
4	Yukon gold potatoes (or other yellow-fleshed variety), peeled and cut into 1-inch (2.5 cm) cubes	4
2	onions, chopped	2
5	large cloves garlic, minced	5
1/2 tsp	saffron threads	2 mL
3	bay leaves	3
3 cups	vegetable stock *or* water	750 mL
1 tbsp	sweet Spanish paprika	15 mL
1 1/2 cups	quartered artichoke hearts (1 can, 14 oz [398 mL])	375 mL
	Salt and freshly ground black pepper	
3 tbsp	fresh parsley	45 mL
	Shaved Parmesan (optional)	
	Lemon wedges (optional)	

1. Soak chickpeas overnight in water to cover or use the quick pressure-soak method, page 130. Drain.

2. In a pressure cooker, heat oil over medium heat. Add potatoes and onions; sauté until onions are tender. Add garlic and saffron; sauté for 1 minute. Stir in chickpeas, bay leaves and stock.

3. Lock the lid in place and bring cooker up to full pressure over high heat. Reduce heat to medium-low, just to maintain even pressure, and cook for 18 minutes. Remove from heat and release pressure quickly.

4. Discard bay leaves. Stir in paprika and artichoke hearts. Simmer, uncovered, over medium heat, breaking up some of the potatoes, until the stew is nicely thickened. Season to taste with salt and pepper. Stir in parsley. If desired, serve with shaved Parmesan and lemon wedges to squeeze over top.

BRAISED SEA BASS PROVENÇAL (PAGE 102) ➤

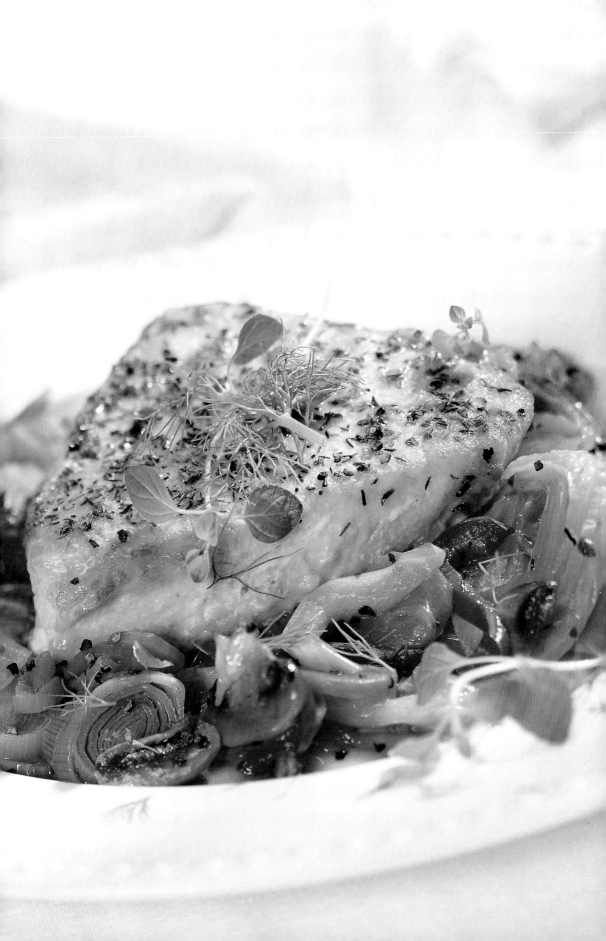

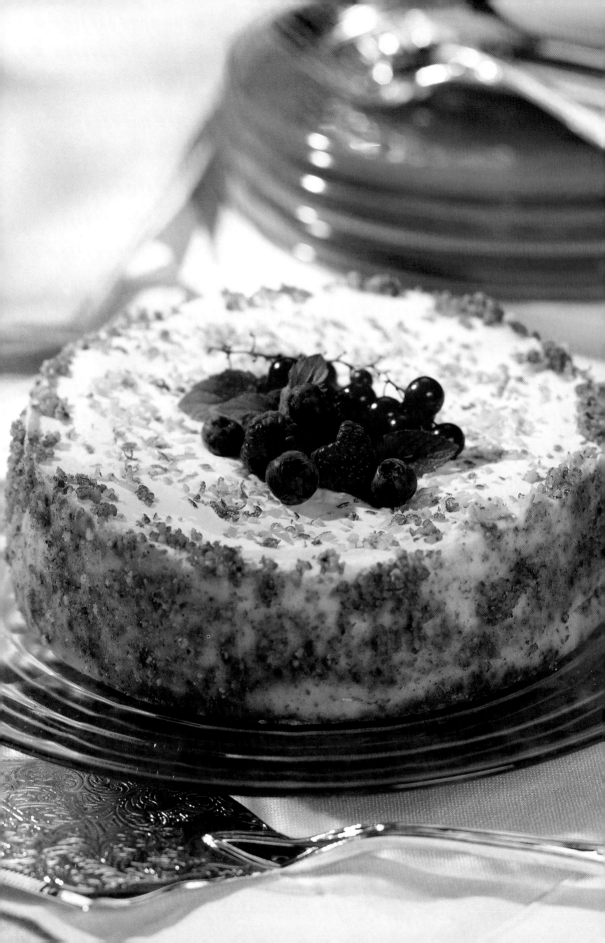

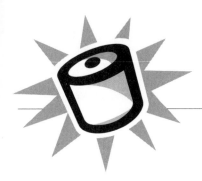

Beans and Grains

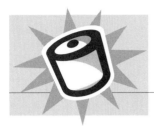

Tips for Preparing Beans

Soaking Methods

All beans need to be soaked before cooking. Soaking rehydrates the beans and helps to remove some of the complex sugars (or oligosaccharides) that give beans a bad name in polite company. There are several procedures for soaking beans which are described below.

TRADITIONAL SOAKING. If you have time, just put your beans in a pot with three or four times their volume in water and let them sit for 4 to 8 hours at room temperature.

QUICK SOAKING. To speed up the soaking process, you can place the beans and water in a pot and bring them to a full, rolling boil. Simmer the beans for 2 minutes, then remove the pot from the heat, cover it, and let the beans soak for 1 hour. Drain away those gaseous complex carbs and proceed with your recipe.

PRESSURE SOAKING. You can speed up the soaking process even further by using the pressure cooker. Place beans and water in pressure cooker (3 cups [750 mL] water for every 1 cup [250 mL] beans, plus 1 tbsp (15 mL) vegetable oil if you have a jiggle-top cooker). Lock the lid in place and bring up to full pressure over high heat. What you do next depends on the size and type of beans you are preparing.

- For small beans, remove the cooker from the heat immediately and let the pressure come down naturally for 10 minutes before releasing remaining steam using the quick-release valve.
- For larger beans, cook under pressure for 1 minute, then allow the pressure to come down naturally for 10 minutes.
- For chickpeas and very large beans, cook for 2 to 3 minutes on high pressure before allowing the pressure to come down naturally for 10 minutes, then releasing any pressure with the quick-release valve.

Checking if beans are fully soaked

The goal of soaking is to have water penetrate to the center of the bean. You can check this by cutting one open to make sure the color is even. An opaque spot in the center indicates the bean needs further soaking, or that you will have to add a few minutes of cooking time while pressure cooking the beans.

Special Precautions for Pressure Cooking Beans and Lentils

If you like legumes or cook a lot of vegetarian dishes, the pressure cooker is a miracle. It allows you to cook inexpensive and healthy dried beans in minutes. Still, there are some precautions to take when you're cooking beans and lentils under pressure.

LEAVE ROOM FOR THE BEANS TO COOK. Make sure you never overload the pressure cooker when cooking beans. Because beans and lentils froth up and expand substantially (up to 4 times their dry size and weight) while cooking, never fill the pressure cooker more than one-third full.

USE ENOUGH WATER. Always use at least 2 cups (500 mL) water or other liquid for every 1 cup (250 mL) dry beans in a recipe. If you have an old-fashioned jiggle-top pressure cooker, always watch it carefully while cooking beans, since the vent can easily become clogged. If it does, you will hear a loud hissing noise. Immediately remove the cooker from the heat and release the pressure. As noted above in the section on soaking beans, jiggle-top pressure cooker users should add 1 tbsp (15 mL) oil to the beans and water before cooking to help reduce foaming and potential clogging.

WATCH YOUR COOKING TIME. Cooking times for beans can vary substantially, depending on a variety of factors, such as the age and dryness of the beans. Even local humidity can affect cooking times. Where a recipe offers a range of cooking times, it's always best to start with the shorter one. You can always finish the beans conventionally or add another minute or two of pressure cooking if they're not quite done. To check for doneness, cut a bean in half with a sharp knife and look at the center. If the beans are done, they will be one color throughout, and tender.

LET PRESSURE DROP NATURALLY. When cooking time is complete, remove the cooker from the heat and allow it to stand until the pressure indicator drops. This helps to avoid clogging the center pipe and safety valve with pulpy cooking liquid. It also prevents the beans from splitting.

KEEP YOUR COOKER CLEAN. Always clean the pressure regulator and lid carefully after cooking beans to make sure there are no obstructions.

NO SALT. Never add salt to a bean recipe before cooking. If you do, the beans can become tough and never really soften properly.

Great Northern Beans Navarre-Style

1 1/2 cups	dried Great Northern beans	375 mL
1 tbsp	olive oil	15 mL
3 tbsp	minced smoky ham or prosciutto	45 mL
3	cloves garlic, minced	3
1	large onion, peeled and chopped	1
1	carrot, finely chopped or grated	1
1	bay leaf	1
1	large plum tomato, seeded and chopped	1
1/4 tsp	freshly ground black pepper	1 mL
4 cups	water	1 L
	Salt to taste	
2 tbsp	chopped parsley	25 mL

Serves 6

This recipe draws its inspiration from Spain, where cooks traditionally use that country's famous *jamon* to flavor the beans. Here we use ham or prosciutto with good results. Serve this savory side dish as an accompaniment to grilled or roasted lamb.

1. Soak beans overnight in water to cover or use the quick pressure-soak method, page 130. Drain.
2. In a pressure cooker, heat oil over medium heat. Add ham, garlic, onion, carrot, bay leaf, tomato and pepper; sauté until vegetables are softened. Stir in beans and water.
3. Lock the lid in place and bring cooker up to full pressure over high heat. Reduce heat to medium-low, just to maintain even pressure, and cook for 10 minutes. Remove from heat and allow pressure to drop naturally. Drain, if necessary.
4. Discard bay leaf. Season to taste with salt and stir in the parsley.

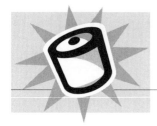

Beans with Shortribs Chuckwagon-Style

Serves 4 to 6

This classic combination was first prepared for me by Alberta rancher Leo Maynard, who won a cooking contest with his tender beef and beans, prepared the old-fashioned way on a wood-fired cook stove. I've speeded up the process considerably using a pressure cooker.

Enjoy this excellent dish as Leo does – with home-made biscuits.

2 cups	dried pinto beans	500 mL
1 tbsp	vegetable oil	15 mL
2 lbs	boneless beef short ribs	1 kg
2	onions, chopped	2
1/4 cup	packed brown sugar	50 mL
1 tbsp	chili powder	15 mL
4 cups	water	1 L
1/2 cup	tomato sauce	125 mL
1 tbsp	prepared mustard	15 mL
2 tsp	cider vinegar	10 mL
1 tsp	Worcestershire sauce	5 mL
1 tsp	liquid smoke	5 mL
1 tsp	salt	5 mL

1. Soak beans overnight in water to cover or use the quick pressure-soak method, page 130. Drain.

2. In a pressure cooker, heat oil over medium-high heat. Add ribs in batches and cook until browned. Transfer to a plate. Set aside.

3. Reduce heat to medium. Add onions and sauté for 10 minutes until tender. Stir in beans, brown sugar, chili powder, water, tomato sauce, mustard, vinegar, Worcestershire and liquid smoke. Place ribs on top.

4. Lock the lid in place and bring cooker up to full pressure over high heat. Reduce heat to medium-low, just to maintain even pressure, and cook for 30 minutes. Remove from heat and release pressure quickly.

5. Stir in salt before serving.

Black Bean Chili

Serves 6 to 8

With earthy black beans, smoky chipotle chilies and a good shot of prairie rye whisky, this is truly an outstanding vegetarian bean dish. Serve it over rice or rolled up in flour tortillas with chopped tomatoes and grated cheese.

2 cups	dried black turtle beans	500 mL
3 tbsp	vegetable oil	45 mL
1	large onion, chopped	1
2 tbsp	paprika	25 mL
1 tbsp	dried oregano	15 mL
2 tsp	cumin seed	10 mL
1/4 tsp	cayenne pepper	1 mL
2	cloves garlic, minced	2
1	chipotle chili in adobo sauce, chopped *or* 1 rehydrated dried chipotle, chopped	1
1	green pepper, chopped	1
1	can (28 oz [796 mL]) plum tomatoes, chopped	1
1	bay leaf	1
1 cup	water	250 mL
1/2 cup	rye whisky	125 mL
2 tsp	salt	10 mL
1/2 cup	chopped cilantro	125 mL
1 cup	grated Cheddar cheese	250 mL
1 cup	sour cream (preferably a low-fat variety)	250 mL

1. Soak beans overnight in water to cover or use the quick pressure-soak method, page 130. Drain.
2. In a pressure cooker, heat oil over medium heat. Add onion and sauté for 5 minutes or until just starting to brown. Add paprika, oregano, cumin and cayenne; cook, stirring constantly, for 2 minutes or just until spices are fragrant. Add garlic, chipotle, green pepper and tomatoes. Stir in beans, bay leaf, water and rye whisky.

3. Lock the lid in place and bring cooker up to full pressure. Reduce heat to medium-low, just to maintain even pressure, and cook for 20 minutes. Remove from heat and allow pressure to drop naturally. The beans should be tender. If not, return to full pressure and cook for 2 to 3 minutes longer. Remove from heat and allow pressure to drop naturally.

4. If beans are too soupy, simmer, uncovered, until reduced and thickened. (Alternatively, transfer 1/2 cup [125 mL] of the beans to a bowl or food processor and mash or purée; stir into the pot.) Discard bay leaf. Season to taste with salt and stir in cilantro. Serve over a mound of fluffy rice, topped with a sprinkling of grated cheese and a dollop of sour cream.

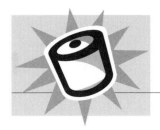

Pork and Beef Chili with Ancho Sauce

Serves 6 to 8

This is a chunky, main-dish chili, packed with tender cubes of meat and earthy black beans.

Ancho chilies are deep-red, medium-hot dried chilies with a rich, sweet flavor that's reminiscent of dried fruit. Chipotle chilies are actually smoked jalapeño chilies. They come dried in packages or packed in adobo sauce in small cans. Both of these special chilies give this dish a complex, smoky flavor that you can't get from fresh chilies alone. Look for them in the produce section of your supermarket, or in specialty grocery stores. If you can't find chipotles, an appropriate substitute is a couple of fresh poblano chilies and a hot jalapeño or serrano chili. You can approximate the chipotle's smokiness by adding a drop of liquid smoke.

1/2 cup	dried black turtle beans	125 mL
2	whole ancho chilies	2
1/4 cup	olive oil	50 mL
1 lb	pork shoulder stew meat, cut into small cubes	500 g
1 lb	beef chuck steak, cut into small cubes	500 g
5	cloves garlic, minced	5
1	large onion, chopped	1
8 oz	spicy Italian sausages, casings removed, meat crumbled	250 g
1 tbsp	ground cumin	15 mL
1 tbsp	red pepper flakes	15 mL
2	cans (19 oz [540 mL]) tomatoes, chopped	2
1/4 cup	rye whisky	50 mL
1 tbsp	dried oregano	15 mL
1 1/2 cups	water	375 mL
1/4 cup	tomato paste	50 mL
	Salt and freshly ground black pepper to taste	

1. Soak beans overnight in water to cover or use the quick pressure-soak method, page 130. Drain. Set aside.
2. In a bowl of hot tap water, soak ancho chilies until softened. Drain and chop, discarding stems and seeds. Set aside.
3. In a pressure cooker, heat oil over medium-high heat. Add pork and beef in batches and cook until browned. Using a slotted spoon, transfer meat to a bowl as it is cooked. Set aside.

4. Add garlic, onion and sausage to cooker; sauté until the onion is softened and sausage is no longer pink. Add red pepper flakes and cumin; sauté for 3 minutes longer. Stir in beans, reserved ancho chilies, pork and beef (with any accumulated juices), oregano, tomatoes, water, rye whisky and tomato paste.

5. Lock the lid in place and bring cooker up to full pressure over high heat. Reduce heat to medium-low, just to maintain even pressure, and cook for 25 minutes. Remove from heat and allow pressure to drop naturally.

6. Season to taste with salt and pepper before serving.

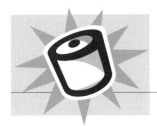

Braised Lima Beans and Bacon

Serves 4

Look for a good butcher where the bacon is double-smoked in-house. The stronger, extra-smoky flavor means that you can use only a small amount of bacon – and therefore add less fat to the dish – without compromising taste.

1 tbsp	olive oil	15 mL
2	slices double-smoked bacon, chopped	2
1	small onion, chopped	1
1	clove garlic, minced	1
1	pkg (1 lb [450 g]) frozen baby lima beans	1
1/2 tsp	freshly ground black pepper	2 mL
1	small plum tomato, chopped	1
1/4 cup	water	50 mL
2 tbsp	chopped parsley	25 mL

1. In a pressure cooker, heat oil over medium-high heat. Add bacon, onion and garlic; sauté until bacon is partly crisp and onion is softened. Stir in lima beans, pepper, tomato and water.

2. Lock the lid in place and bring cooker up to full pressure over high heat. Reduce heat to medium-low, just to maintain even pressure, and cook for 10 minutes. Remove from heat and release pressure quickly. Stir in parsley. Serve immediately.

Campfire Beans with Cheese

Serves 6

This fast and easy dish makes a healthy alternative to mac and cheese that kids love. For adult tastes, you can torque up the spice with more hot sauce at the table.

2 cups	dried pinto beans	500 mL
1	ham hock or ham bone	1
1	onion, peeled, whole	1
4 cups	water	1 L
3 tbsp	butter	45 mL
8 oz	old Cheddar cheese, grated	250 g
1 cup	finely chopped onions	250 mL
2	cloves garlic, minced	2
1 to 2 tsp	hot sauce (Prairie Fire, Tabasco, Durkee's or other hot sauce)	5 to 10 mL
	Salt and freshly ground black pepper to taste	

1. Soak beans overnight in water to cover or use the quick pressure-soak method, page 130. Drain.

2. In a pressure cooker, combine beans, ham hock, whole onion and water. Lock the lid in place and bring cooker up to full pressure over high heat. Reduce heat to medium-low, just to maintain even pressure, and cook for 10 minutes. Remove from heat and allow pressure to drop naturally.

3. Drain, reserving liquid. Discard onion. Remove hock; cut away any meat from bone, chop and set aside. Discard bone and scraps. Return meat and beans to cooker; stir in butter, cheese, minced onions, garlic and hot sauce to taste. Stir to combine well, adding enough of the reserved cooking liquid to make a creamy sauce. Warm gently over low heat until cheese melts; simmer just until everything is tender. Season with salt and pepper to taste. Serve with hot sauce.

Mushroom, Italian Sausage and Braised Lentil Stew

Serves 4

Serve this savory lentil stew over rice (or short pasta such as orecchiette or rotini) for a fast, healthy supper.

TIP

Beans and lentils tend to froth up in a pressure cooker, so make sure the cooker is no more than one-third full. If there's too much of this stew for your pot, cook it in two batches, cleaning the pressure release valve carefully after cooking each batch.

1 lb	mild or spicy fresh Italian sausage, casings removed, meat crumbled	500 g
1 to 2 tbsp	olive oil	15 to 25 mL
2	stalks celery, chopped	2
2	cloves garlic, minced	2
1	large onion, chopped	1
1 cup	chopped mushrooms	250 mL
1	carrot, minced	1
2 cups	small French green lentils	500 mL
3	plum tomatoes, chopped	3
1/2 tsp	dried thyme	2 mL
1/2 tsp	dried sage	2 mL
3 cups	chicken stock	750 mL
1 cup	dry red wine	250 mL
	Salt and freshly ground black pepper	
2 tbsp	chopped basil *or* basil pesto	25 mL
	Cooked brown rice or short pasta (orecchiette, rotini, penne)	

1. In a pressure cooker, heat 1 tbsp (15 mL) of the oil over medium-high heat. Add sausage and cook until browned. Transfer to a bowl. Set aside.

2. Reduce heat to medium; add more oil if necessary to prevent burning. Add celery, garlic, onion and mushrooms; sauté for 5 minutes or until vegetables are soft and beginning to color. Add lentils, tomatoes, thyme, sage, 1/4 tsp (1 mL) salt, 1/4 tsp (1 mL) pepper, stock and wine. Stir in cooked sausage.

3. Lock the lid in place and bring cooker up to full pressure over high heat. Reduce heat to medium-low, just to maintain even pressure, and cook for 8 minutes. Remove from heat and allow pressure to drop naturally.

4. Simmer, uncovered, to reduce any excess liquid in the pot. Stir in basil and season to taste with salt and pepper. Serve over rice or pasta.

Wheat Berries Carbonara

2 cups	whole wheat berries *or* whole grain rye	500 mL
1 tsp	salt	5 mL
6 cups	water	1.5 L
3 tbsp	olive oil, divided	45 mL
2	onions, finely chopped	2
8 oz	Canadian back bacon, slivered	250 g
1 cup	frozen peas, thawed	250 mL
1 cup	whipping (35%) cream	250 mL
1 cup	freshly grated Parmesan cheese	250 mL
	Salt and freshly ground black pepper to taste	

Serves 4

Here's a great way to enjoy the flavors of a creamy Italian sauce with a healthy serving of whole grain.

TIP

Substitute whole raw buckwheat for wheat berries; reduce water to 4 cups (1 L) and cooking time to 15 minutes.

1. In a pressure cooker, combine wheat berries, salt, water and 1 tbsp (15 mL) of the oil. Lock the lid in place and bring cooker up to full pressure over high heat. Reduce heat to medium-low, just to maintain even pressure, and cook for 35 to 40 minutes. Remove from heat and release pressure quickly. The wheat berries should be tender. If not, return to full pressure and cook for 3 to 5 minutes longer. Remove from heat and release pressure quickly. Drain well.

2. Meanwhile, in a large sauté pan, heat the remaining oil over medium-high heat. Add onions and bacon; sauté until onions are golden brown. Add peas and heat through. Stir in cream and cooked wheat berries, stirring to coat.

3. Reduce heat to medium-low and cook just until heated through. Stir in Parmesan cheese. Season to taste with salt and pepper. Serve immediately.

Basic Risotto

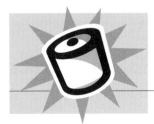

Serves 4 as a side dish

The pressure cooker makes cooking creamy risotto so easy, you'll be serving it instead of regular rice all the time. The saffron is optional, but it gives the risotto a wonderful earthy flavor and golden color. A wood rasp makes an excellent grater for the Parmesan.

TIP

Use homemade chicken stock (see recipe, page 175) for the best flavor. Otherwise, use a good-quality commercially prepared stock.

1 tbsp	butter	15 mL
1 tbsp	olive oil	15 mL
1	small onion, minced	1
1 cup	Arborio rice *or* other short-grain rice	250 mL
1/4 cup	dry white wine	50 mL
2 cups	chicken stock *or* vegetable stock	500 mL
1/2 tsp	crushed saffron threads (optional)	2 mL
1/2 cup	freshly grated Parmesan cheese	125 mL
	Freshly ground black pepper	

1. In a pressure cooker, heat butter and oil over medium heat. Add onion and sauté for 5 minutes until soft (but not brown). Stir in rice, coating well with oil. Add wine. If using, crumble saffron into stock. Pour stock over rice.

2. Lock the lid in place and bring cooker up to full pressure over high heat. Reduce heat to medium-low, just to maintain even pressure, and cook for 7 minutes. Remove from heat and release pressure quickly. Stir in Parmesan cheese and season to taste with pepper. Serve immediately.

Risotto with Mushrooms and Shrimp

Serves 2 as a main dish or 4 as a side dish

The pressure cooker is brilliant for risotto – the creamy rice dish cooks by itself in 6 to 7 minutes. This version makes an elegant dinner for two with a salad to start, or a great first course for four.

TIP

Use homemade chicken stock (see recipe, page 175) for the best flavor. Otherwise, use a good-quality commercially prepared stock.

2 tbsp	olive oil	25 mL
1 tbsp	butter	15 mL
2	cloves garlic, minced	2
1 cup	sliced mixed mushrooms (such as brown, oyster, portobello, shiitake, morel)	250 mL
1	onion, sliced	1
1 tsp	chopped thyme	5 mL
1 cup	Arborio rice *or* other short-grain rice	250 mL
2 cups	chicken stock	500 mL
1/4 cup	dry white wine	50 mL
12 oz	medium to large shrimp, peeled, deveined and cut in half lengthwise	375 g
1/2 cup	freshly grated Parmesan cheese	125 mL

1. In a pressure cooker, heat oil and butter over medium heat. Add garlic, mushrooms and onion; sauté for 5 minutes or until softened (but not brown). Stir in thyme and rice; sauté for 1 minute. Pour in stock and wine.

2. Lock the lid in place and bring cooker up to full pressure over high heat. Reduce heat to medium-low, just to maintain even pressure, and cook for 7 minutes. Remove from heat and release pressure quickly.

3. Stir in the shrimp; cover (but do not lock) and let stand for 10 minutes until shrimp are opaque. Stir in the Parmesan. Serve immediately.

Risotto with Grilled Vegetables and Beet Greens

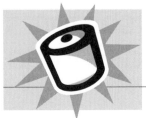

Serves 4

Loaded with grilled vegetables and healthy greens, this risotto may be served as a vegetarian main course.

TIP

Use homemade chicken stock (see recipe, page 175) for the best flavor. Otherwise, use a good-quality commercially prepared stock.

1/4 cup	extra virgin olive oil	50 mL
1	clove garlic, minced	1
1	small Asian eggplant, sliced	1
1	small zucchini, sliced	1
1	portobello mushroom, stem removed	1
1	red or yellow bell pepper, seeded and halved	1
1	onion, thickly sliced	1
	Salt and freshly ground black pepper to taste	
1/4 cup	butter, divided	50 mL
1 cup	Arborio rice *or* other short-grain rice	250 mL
1/2 cup	dry white wine	125 mL
2 cups	chicken stock	500 mL
2 cups	slivered young beet greens	500 mL
1/4 cup	slivered basil leaves	50 mL
1/2 cup	freshly grated Parmesan cheese	125 mL

1. In a small bowl, combine oil and garlic; let stand at room temperature for 10 minutes to infuse flavor. Brush over the eggplant, zucchini, mushroom, bell pepper and onion. Season with salt and pepper. Grill over medium heat, turning once, until softened and slightly charred. Let cool. Chop coarsely and set aside.

2. In a pressure cooker, heat 3 tbsp (45 mL) of the butter with any of the remaining oil and garlic over medium heat. Add rice, stirring to coat. Stir in stock and wine.

3. Lock the lid in place and bring cooker up to full pressure over high heat. Reduce heat to medium-low, just to maintain even pressure, and cook for 7 minutes. Remove from heat and release pressure quickly.

4. Stir in grilled vegetables, beet greens and basil. Cover (but do not lock) and let stand just until the greens are wilted, about 5 minutes. Stir in Parmesan cheese and remaining butter; season to taste with pepper.

Roasted Garlic Risotto with Asiago

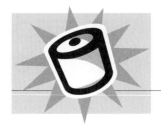

Serves 4 to 6

Roasting tames the natural harshness of garlic and gives it a buttery, nutty flavor that works perfectly with the strong cheese in this dish. The lemon zest adds sparkle; the green onion, a touch of color. There's nothing complicated about this risotto, and it demonstrates once again just how easy it is to make a spectacular side dish in 7 short minutes.

PREHEAT OVEN TO 350° F (180° C)

1	head garlic	1
1 tsp	olive oil	5 mL
3 tbsp	butter	45 mL
1	large onion, finely chopped	1
2 cups	Arborio rice *or* other short-grain rice	500 mL
1/2 cup	dry white wine	50 mL
4 cups	chicken stock	500 mL
1 cup	freshly grated Asiago cheese	250 mL
1/4 cup	minced green onions	50 mL
1 tsp	minced lemon zest	5 mL
	Freshly ground black pepper to taste	

1. To roast garlic, cut top quarter-inch from whole head to expose cloves; drizzle with oil and wrap loosely in foil. Roast in preheated oven for 30 to 40 minutes, until garlic is very soft. Press roasted garlic out of skins and mash with the flat side of a knife. Set aside.

2. In a pressure cooker, heat butter over medium heat. Add onion and sauté for 5 minutes, until soft (but not brown). Add rice, stirring to coat. Stir in the wine and cook until it has been absorbed. Stir in reserved garlic and chicken stock.

3. Lock the lid in place and bring cooker up to full pressure over high heat. Reduce heat to medium-low, just to maintain even pressure, and cook for 7 minutes. Remove from heat and release pressure quickly.

4. Stir in cheese, green onions and lemon zest. Season to taste with pepper. Serve immediately.

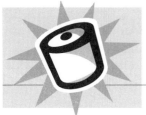

Barley with Mint and Root Vegetables

Serves 6

Barley is a healthy whole grain that makes a nice substitute for rice. Prepared in the pressure cooker, it's fast, tooth-some and never sticky.

Adding grated Parmesan to this dish gives it a flavor that's reminiscent of risotto.

Be sure to caramelize the vegetables until they're nice and brown – that's what gives this savory root vegetable dish it a full, rich flavor.

1/4 cup	butter	50 mL
2	carrots, cut into small cubes	2
2	parsnips, cut into small cubes	2
1	sweet potato, peeled and cubed	1
1	onion, chopped	1
1 cup	pot or pearl barley	250 mL
3	cloves garlic, minced	3
3 cups	chicken *or* brown stock	750 mL
2 tbsp	chopped mint	25 mL
2 tbsp	chopped parsley (optional)	25 mL
1 cup	finely grated Parmesan or Asiago cheese (optional)	250 mL
	Salt and freshly ground black pepper to taste	

1. In a pressure cooker, heat butter over medium heat. Add carrots, parsnips, sweet potato and onion; sauté until vegetables start to caramelize. Add barley and garlic; cook, stirring, for 5 minutes to toast the grains. Pour in stock.

2. Lock the lid in place and bring cooker up to full pressure over high heat. Reduce heat to medium-low, just to maintain even pressure, and cook for 20 minutes. Remove from heat and release pressure quickly. The barley should be tender. If not, cover (but do not lock) and simmer over low heat until tender.

3. Stir in mint, parsley and Parmesan (if using). Season to taste with salt and pepper.

Indian Rice Pilau

Serves 4 as a side dish

Here's the perfect rice dish to accompany ROGAN JOSH (see recipe, page 82) or, for vegetarians, CURRIED LENTILS WITH SPINACH (see recipe, page 127). The brown basmati gives extra flavor and fiber, but takes a little longer to cook than regular rice. For extra color and crunch, finish this dish by adding your choice of raisins, currants, chopped red bell pepper or green onions.

1/4 cup	butter	50 mL
1	small onion, minced	1
4	green cardamom pods	4
1	cinnamon stick	1
1	bay leaf	1
1/2 tsp	ground turmeric	2 mL
1/2 tsp	ground cumin	2 mL
1 1/2 cups	brown basmati rice	375 mL
1/2 tsp	salt	2 mL
2 cups	water *or* vegetable stock	500 mL
1/2 cup	raisins *or* currants *and/or* finely chopped red bell pepper and green onions to finish (optional)	125 mL

1. In a pressure cooker, heat butter over medium heat. Add onion, cardamom, cinnamon, bay leaf, turmeric and cumin; sauté until onion is soft and spices are fragrant. Add rice, stirring to coat. Add salt and water; bring to a boil.

2. Lock the lid in place and bring cooker up to full pressure over high heat. Reduce heat to medium-low, just to maintain even pressure, and cook for 9 minutes. Remove from heat and allow pressure to drop naturally for 7 to 10 minutes. Release any remaining pressure quickly.

3. Fluff rice with a fork; discard cinnamon stick and bay leaf. If desired, stir in raisins, currants, red pepper or green onions.

Wild Rice Casserole with Mixed Mushrooms and Chestnuts

Serves 4

This side dish makes a great addition to Thanksgiving or Christmas dinner. You can also use it as a stuffing for roast chicken, game hens – even whole baked salmon. For an interesting flavor variation, and to accompany richer meats such as goose or duck, try replacing the mushrooms with dried fruits such as currants, apricots or cranberries.

TIP

The pressure cooker makes peeling chestnuts fast and easy. Cut an X in the base of each nut and place in the cooker; cover nuts with plenty of water, lock lid in place, and cook at high pressure for 6 minutes. You'll find it's easy to peel off the shells and the brown, papery skin (which is bitter).

You can also use your pressure cooker to speed-soak the smoky-flavored dried chestnuts sold in Italian and Asian markets throughout the year. Allow 2 minutes of cooking under pressure and 10 minutes of natural pressure release to rehydrate the dried chestnuts.

2 tbsp	butter	25 mL
1	onion, finely chopped	1
2	cloves garlic, minced	2
1 cup	sliced mixed mushrooms (such as portobello, oyster, shiitake and white)	250 mL
1 cup	wild rice	250 mL
1 cup	cooked and crumbled chestnuts *or* 1/2 cup (125 mL) toasted pecans	250 mL
2	sprigs thyme (or 1 tsp [5 mL] dried)	2
2 cups	chicken stock	500 mL
	Salt and freshly ground black pepper to taste	

1. In a pressure cooker, melt butter over medium heat. Add garlic, onion and mushrooms; sauté until they start to brown. Stir in wild rice, chestnuts, thyme and stock. Bring to a boil.

2. Lock the lid in place and bring cooker up to full pressure over high heat. Reduce heat to medium-low, just to maintain even pressure, and cook for 20 minutes. Remove from heat and allow pressure to drop naturally. The rice should be tender, with many of the grains broken and curled. If not, return to full pressure and cook for 2 to 3 minutes longer. Remove from heat and allow pressure to drop naturally.

3. Drain off any excess liquid. Discard thyme sprigs. Season to taste with salt and pepper.

Desserts

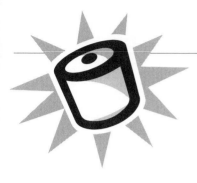

Lemon-Lime Cheesecake

7- OR 8-INCH (1.5 OR 2 L) SPRINGFORM PAN (USE SMALLER SIZE IF NECESSARY TO FIT INSIDE PRESSURE COOKER)
RACK OR TRIVET TO FIT BOTTOM OF PRESSURE COOKER

Serves 6 to 8

This classic, dense, citrusy cheesecake is wonderful served with a fresh or lightly cooked fruit sauce. Try it topped with Saskatoon or blueberries that have been simmered with a little water and sugar, or drizzle with a tart lemon syrup made by boiling 1/4 cup (50 mL) fresh lemon juice with 1/3 cup (75 mL) sugar for a couple of minutes, then chilling.

TIP

Cheesecake can be wrapped and refrigerated for up to 3 days or frozen for up to 3 months.

CRUST

3 tbsp	butter, softened	45 mL
3 tbsp	crushed vanilla wafers	45 mL
3 tbsp	ground pecans	45 mL

FILLING

	Zest and juice of 1 lemon	
	Zest and juice of 1 lime	
1 lb	cream cheese	500 g
1 cup	granulated sugar	250 mL
3 tbsp	all-purpose flour	45 mL
4	eggs	4
1/4 cup	plain yogurt *or* sour cream	50 mL
1 tsp	vanilla extract	5 mL
2 cups	water for steaming	500 mL

TOPPING

1/2 cup	sour cream	125 mL
2 tbsp	granulated sugar	25 mL
	Mixed fresh fruit and berries for topping (sliced peaches, blueberries, sliced strawberries, etc.)	

1. CRUST: Thickly butter the bottom and sides of springform pan. In a bowl combine crushed wafers and pecans; sprinkle inside pan, tilting to coat sides. Leave excess crumbs on bottom. Wrap outside of pan with foil to seal. Set aside.

2. In a bowl combine lemon zest and lime zest. Reserve 1 tsp (5 mL), covered and refrigerated, for garnish.

3. FILLING: In a food processor, purée remaining lemon and lime zest together with lemon juice, lime juice, cream cheese, sugar and flour. With motor running, add eggs one at a time. Add yogurt and vanilla; purée for 10 seconds or until smooth. Pour into prepared pan and cover with a piece of buttered foil, making sure pan is well sealed.

4. Set rack in bottom of pressure cooker. Pour in water. Fold a two-foot (60 cm) long piece of foil several times to make a strip that will be used to remove pan. Center pan on midpoint of strip and fold the ends together to make a handle. Use strip to lower pan into the cooker.

5. Lock the lid in place and bring cooker up to full pressure over high heat. Reduce heat to medium-low, just to maintain even pressure, and cook for 20 minutes. Remove from heat and allow pressure to drop naturally for 7 minutes. Release remaining pressure quickly. Let cheesecake cool in cooker for a few minutes. Using foil handle, lift pan out of cooker onto cooling rack. Remove foil lid. Cheesecake should be set around edges, but still slightly loose in center. If center is still liquid, seal with foil and return to cooker. Bring up to full pressure and cook for 2 minutes longer. Remove from heat and allow pressure to drop as above. When cheesecake is cooked, remove foil. Use a paper towel to mop up any water pooled on top of cake.

6. TOPPING: In a small bowl, whisk sour cream with sugar. Spread over cheesecake, smoothing top. Let cool to room temperature. Refrigerate for at least 8 hours or overnight before serving.

7. Serve garnished with fresh fruit and sprinkle with reserved zest.

Layered White and Dark Chocolate Cheesecake

7- OR 8-INCH (1.5 OR 2 L) SPRINGFORM PAN (USE SMALLER SIZE IF NECESSARY TO FIT INSIDE PRESSURE COOKER)
RACK OR TRIVET TO FIT BOTTOM OF PRESSURE COOKER

Serves 6 to 8

What could be more tempting than your favorite dark- and white-chocolate cheesecakes – together? The layers look lovely and you can top the whole thing with a decadent layer of sweet-ened sour cream (which also masks any cracks that may have formed in the top of your cake during cooking).

TIP

Cheesecake can be wrapped and refrigerated for up to 3 days or frozen for up to 3 months.

CRUST

2 tbsp	butter, softened	25 mL
1/4 cup	chocolate cookie crumbs	50 mL

FILLING

2 oz	semi-sweet chocolate, chopped	50 g
2 oz	white chocolate, chopped	50 g
1 lb	cream cheese	500 g
1/2 cup	granulated sugar	125 mL
2 tbsp	all-purpose flour	25 mL
4	eggs	4
1/2 cup	sour cream *or* yogurt	125 mL
1/2 tsp	vanilla extract	2 mL
2 cups	water for steaming	500 mL

TOPPING

1/2 cup	sour cream	125 mL
2 tbsp	granulated sugar	25 mL
	Fresh strawberries	

1. CRUST: Thickly butter bottom and sides of springform pan. Sprinkle cookie crumbs inside pan, tilting to coat sides. Leave excess crumbs on bottom. Wrap outside of pan with foil to seal. Set aside.

2. FILLING: In a heatproof bowl set over hot (not boiling) water, melt semi-sweet chocolate. In a separate bowl, melt white chocolate. Let both chocolates cool slightly.

3. In a food processor, purée cream cheese, sugar and flour. With motor running, add eggs one at a time. Add sour cream and vanilla; purée for 10 seconds or until smooth. Divide batter evenly between the two bowls of melted chocolate. Stir both to combine well. Pour dark chocolate filling into prepared crust. Gently pour white chocolate filling over top. Cover with a piece of buttered foil, making sure pan is well sealed.

4. Set rack in the bottom of pressure cooker. Pour in water. Fold a two-foot (60 cm) long piece of foil several times to make a strip that will be used to remove pan. Center pan on midpoint of strip and fold the ends together to make a handle. Use strip to lower pan into the cooker.

5. Lock the lid in place and bring cooker up to full pressure over high heat. Reduce heat to medium-low, just to maintain even pressure, and cook for 20 minutes. Remove from heat and allow pressure to drop naturally for 7 minutes. Release remaining pressure quickly. Let cheesecake cool in cooker for a few minutes. Using foil handle, lift pan out of cooker onto cooling rack. Remove foil lid. Cheesecake should be set around edges, but still slightly loose in center. If center is still liquid, seal with foil and return to cooker. Bring up to full pressure and cook for 2 minutes longer. Remove from heat and allow pressure to drop as above. When cheesecake is cooked, remove foil. Use a paper towel to mop up any water pooled on top of cake.

6. TOPPING: In a small bowl, whisk sour cream with sugar. Spread over cheesecake, smoothing top. Let cool to room temperature. Refrigerate for at least 8 hours or overnight before serving.

7. Serve garnished with strawberries.

Orange Espresso Cheesecake

7- OR 8-INCH (1.5 OR 2 L) SPRINGFORM PAN (USE SMALLER SIZE
IF NECESSARY TO FIT INSIDE PRESSURE COOKER)
RACK OR TRIVET TO FIT BOTTOM OF PRESSURE COOKER

Serves 6 to 8

It's still amazing to me
that cheesecake "bakes"
far better in a pressure
cooker than it does in the
oven. But the high tem-
perature and steam result
in a cake that's infinitely
creamier and has less
crust (and therefore far
less fat). It's a winning
method – try it.

TIP

Cheesecake can be
wrapped and refrigerated
for up to 3 days or frozen
for up to 3 months.

CRUST

3 tbsp	butter, softened	45 mL
1/3 cup	graham wafer crumbs	75 mL

FILLING

	Zest and juice of 1 large navel orange (about 1/2 cup [125 mL] juice)	
1 lb	cream cheese	500 g
1 cup	granulated sugar	250 mL
3 tbsp	all-purpose flour	45 mL
2 tbsp	instant espresso	25 mL
1/4 cup	warm water	50 mL
1/4 tsp	ground cloves	1 mL
1/2 tsp	ground cinnamon	2 mL
2 tbsp	Grand Marnier *or* 1 tbsp (25 mL) brandy and 1 tbsp (15mL)Triple Sec	25 mL
4	eggs	4
2 cups	water for steaming	500 mL

TOPPING

1/2 cup	sour cream	125 mL
2 tbsp	granulated sugar	25 mL
1 tbsp	Grand Marnier or Triple Sec	15 mL
	Fresh orange segments for garnish	

1. CRUST: Thickly butter bottom and sides of springform
   pan. Sprinkle graham crumbs inside pan, tilting to coat
   sides. Leave excess crumbs on bottom. Wrap outside of
   pan with foil to seal. Set aside.

2. FILLING: Wrap and refrigerate 1 tsp (5 mL) of the orange zest for garnish. In a small bowl, dissolve the instant espresso in the warm water.

3. In a food processor, purée remaining orange zest, orange juice, cream cheese, sugar and flour until smooth. Add espresso mixture, cloves, cinnamon and Grand Marnier; purée until smooth. With motor running, add eggs one at a time and purée for another 10 seconds, until well combined. Cover with a piece of buttered foil, making sure pan is well sealed.

4. Set rack in the bottom of pressure cooker. Pour in water. Fold a two-foot (60 cm) long piece of foil several times to make a strip that will be used to remove pan. Center pan on midpoint of strip and fold the ends together to make a handle. Use strip to lower pan into the cooker.

5. Lock the lid in place and bring cooker up to full pressure over high heat. Reduce heat to medium-low, just to maintain even pressure, and cook for 20 minutes. Remove from heat and allow pressure to drop naturally for 7 minutes. Release remaining pressure quickly. Let cheesecake cool in cooker for a few minutes. Using foil handle, lift pan out of cooker onto cooling rack. Remove foil lid. Cheesecake should be set around edges, but still slightly loose in center. If center is still liquid, seal with foil and return to cooker. Bring up to full pressure and cook for 2 minutes longer. Remove from heat and allow pressure to drop as above. When cheesecake is cooked, remove foil. Use a paper towel to mop up any water pooled on top of cake.

6. TOPPING: In a small bowl, whisk together sour cream and sugar. Spread over cheesecake, smoothing top. Let cool to room temperature. Refrigerate for at least 8 hours or overnight before serving.

7. Sprinkle cheesecake with reserved orange zest and serve with orange segments.

Coconut Crème Caramel

6-CUP (1.5 L) SOUFFLÉ DISH (USE SMALLER SIZE IF NECESSARY TO FIT INSIDE PRESSURE COOKER)

RACK OR TRIVET TO FIT BOTTOM OF PRESSURE COOKER

Serves 8

This variation on a classic dessert makes the perfect ending to a spicy Thai or Szechuan meal. Serve it with slices of ripe mango, papaya and star fruit, or a drizzle of passion fruit coulis

1 cup	granulated sugar	250 mL
2 1/4 cups	water, divided	550 mL
1 cup	milk	250 mL
1	can (14 oz [398 mL]) coconut milk	1
1	can (10 oz [300 mL]) low-fat sweetened condensed milk	1
1/2 tsp	vanilla extract	2 mL
3	eggs	3
2	egg yolks	2

Sliced tropical fruits for garnish
(such as papaya, mango, star fruit, etc.)

TIP

If you wish to make individual puddings, use eight 1/2-cup (125 mL) straight-sided soufflé dishes; wrap each well with foil after filling and stack on the trivet or in the steamer basket of your pressure cooker. These smaller crème caramels need only about 12 minutes under pressure. Let pressure drop naturally after steaming, then chill for several hours. The puddings can be turned out on individual dessert dishes for serving.

1. In a saucepan combine sugar and 1/4 cup (50 mL) of the water. Bring to a boil, without stirring, over medium-high heat. Continue to boil, swirling pan occasionally to prevent burning, for about 7 minutes or until syrup is a deep caramel colour. Carefully pour into soufflé dish, swirling to coat bottom and sides with caramel. Set aside.

2. In another saucepan, whisk together milk, coconut milk and condensed milk. Heat over medium heat until bubbles form around edge of pan and mixture is steaming. Stir in vanilla. In a bowl whisk eggs together with egg yolks. Whisk in a little of the hot milk mixture. Gradually whisk egg-milk mixture back into saucepan. Cook over low heat, stirring constantly, for about 4 minutes or until mixture is slightly thickened. Do not boil. Pour into soufflé dish; cover with a piece of foil, making sure dish is well sealed.

3. Set rack in the bottom of pressure cooker. Pour in remaining water. Fold a two-foot (60 cm) long piece of foil several times to make a strip that will be used to remove dish. Center dish on midpoint of strip and fold the ends together to make a handle. Use strip to lower dish into the cooker.

4. Lock the lid in place and bring cooker up to full pressure over high heat. Reduce heat to medium-low, just to maintain even pressure, and cook for 30 minutes. Remove from heat and allow pressure to drop naturally for 30 minutes. Using foil handle, lift dish out of cooker onto cooling rack. Remove foil lid. The custard should be just set in the middle. If center is still loose, seal with foil and return to cooker. Bring up to full pressure and cook for 2 minutes longer. Remove from heat and allow pressure to drop as above. When custard is cooked, remove foil.

5. Let cool to room temperature. Cover with plastic wrap and chill for at least 12 hours or for up to 24 hours. To serve, run a sharp knife around edge of caramel to loosen. Invert on a rimmed plate. Slice into wedges and garnish with fresh fruit.

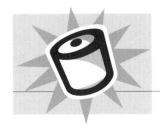

Classic Christmas Plum Pudding

Serves 8 to 10

This is the only way to produce a plum pudding – moist and ready so fast, you'll never steam your Christmas pudding in a conventional steamer again!

You can use a 6-cup (1.5 L) heatproof bowl or pudding mold that fits easily into your pressure cooker to make the classic-shaped holiday pudding, but the pudding cooks most evenly in a 7- to 8-inch (17.5 to 20 cm) springform pan or ring mold.

While this dense fruit pudding can be prepared and eaten on the same day, it's best made in advance and refrigerated for 2 to 4 weeks, wrapped in a brandy-soaked cheesecloth. You can then re-steam the pudding for 10 minutes in the pressure cooker or reheat it in the microwave before serving with the warm brandy sauce. Happy holidays!

7- OR 8-INCH (1.5 OR 2 L) SPRINGFORM PAN (*OR* HEATPROOF BOWL *OR* PUDDING MOLD), BUTTERED (USE SMALLER SIZE IF NECESSARY TO FIT INSIDE PRESSURE COOKER)

RACK OR TRIVET TO FIT BOTTOM OF PRESSURE COOKER

2 cups	dried currants	500 mL
1 cup	dark raisins	250 mL
1 cup	dried cranberries	250 mL
1 cup	minced candied lemon peel *or* citron	250 mL
1/2 cup	brandy *or* rum	125 mL
1 1/2 cups	all-purpose flour	375 mL
1 cup	bread crumbs	250 mL
1/2 cup	chopped pecans	125 mL
1 tbsp	chopped candied ginger	15 mL
1 tsp	baking soda	5 mL
1 tsp	ground cinnamon	5 mL
1/2 tsp	salt	2 mL
1/4 tsp	ground nutmeg	1 mL
1/4 tsp	ground cloves	1 mL
3/4 cup	butter, very cold or partially frozen	175 mL
1 cup	packed brown sugar	250 mL
3	eggs	3
3 cups	water for steaming	750 mL

BRANDY SAUCE

1 cup	packed brown sugar	250 mL
1 cup	whipping (35%) cream	250 mL
1/4 cup	butter	50 mL
1/4 cup	brandy *or* rum	50 mL

1. In a bowl combine currants, raisins, dried cranberries, candied lemon peel and brandy. Cover and let stand at room temperature for 8 hours.

2. In a large bowl, combine flour, breadcrumbs, pecans, ginger, baking soda, cinnamon, salt, nutmeg and cloves. Using a cheese grater, grate butter into bowl; add marinated fruit. With your hands, toss to mix. In a separate bowl, beat eggs together with brown sugar; pour over the batter. Using hands, combine well.

3. Wrap base of springform pan with foil and pack the batter into pan, pressing to eliminate any air pockets. Cover with a piece of buttered foil, making sure pan is well sealed. Use kitchen string to tie foil tightly in place.

4. Set rack in the bottom of pressure cooker. Pour in water. Fold a two-foot (60 cm) long piece of foil several times to make a strip that will be used to remove pan. Center pan on midpoint of strip and fold the ends together to make a handle. Use strip to lower pan into the cooker.

5. Lock the lid in place and bring cooker up to full pressure over high heat. Reduce heat to medium-low, just to maintain even pressure, and cook for 1 hour. Remove from heat and allow pressure to drop naturally. Using foil handle, lift pan out of cooker onto cooling rack. Remove foil lid. Let cool for 15 minutes. Run a sharp knife around edge of pudding to loosen and unmold onto a plate. Let cool to lukewarm.

6. BRANDY SAUCE: In a saucepan over medium-low heat, combine brown sugar, cream, butter and brandy. Simmer, stirring, for about 10 minutes or until sauce coats the back of a spoon. Serve pudding warm with brandy sauce.

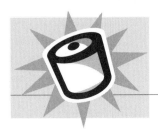

Apricot Bread-and-Butter Pudding with Brandy Cream

6- TO 8-CUP (1.5 TO 2 L) SOUFFLÉ DISH (USE SMALLER SIZE IF NECESSARY TO FIT INSIDE PRESSURE COOKER)

RACK OR TRIVET TO FIT BOTTOM OF PRESSURE COOKER

Serves 8 to 10

Dried winter fruits and brandy add a unique flavor to this rich and comforting dessert. Make it in a 6- to 8-cup (1.5 to 2 L) soufflé dish that will fit easily into your pressure cooker.

PUDDING

1/2 cup	dried apricots, slivered	125 mL
1/2 cup	raisins	125 mL
1/2 cup	slivered almonds	125 mL
1/2 cup	pecans, toasted	125 mL
1/4 cup	diced candied orange peel	50 mL
1/2 cup	melted butter	125 mL
1	large loaf of dense white bread, sliced, crusts removed	1
	Brown sugar	
4	eggs	4
3/4 cup	granulated sugar	175 mL
1/2 tsp	ground nutmeg	2 mL
1 tsp	ground cinnamon	5 mL
1 cup	milk	250 mL
2 tbsp	cognac *or* rum	25 mL
1 tbsp	vanilla extract	15 mL

BRANDY CREAM SAUCE

1 cup	whipping (35%) cream	250 mL
1/2 cup	2% milk	125 mL
1/4 tsp	vanilla extract	1 mL
1/4 cup	granulated sugar	50 mL
Pinch	salt	Pinch
3	egg yolks	3
1/2 cup	brandy	125 mL

1. PUDDING: In a bowl combine apricots, raisins, almonds, pecans and orange peel. Set aside.   *(Recipe continues...)*

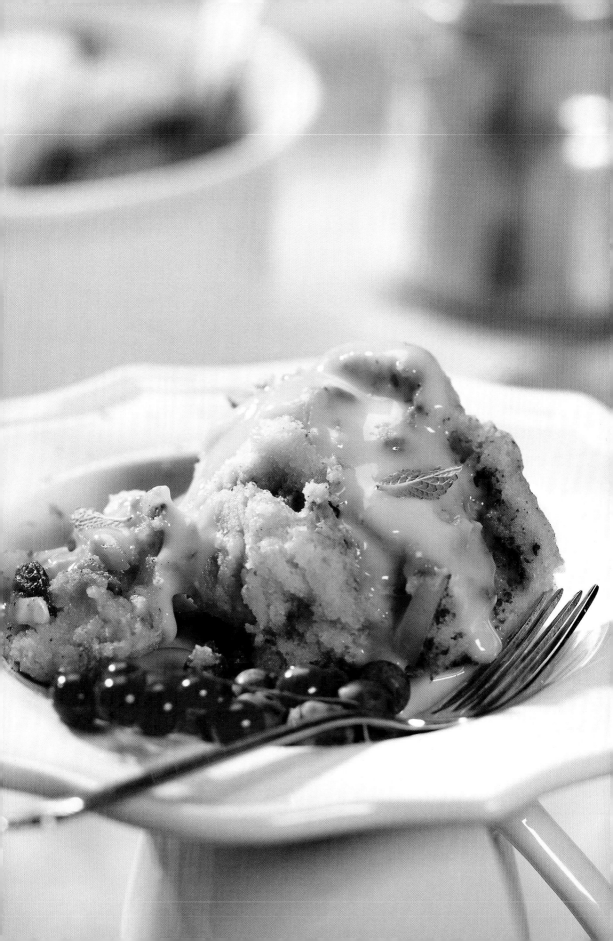

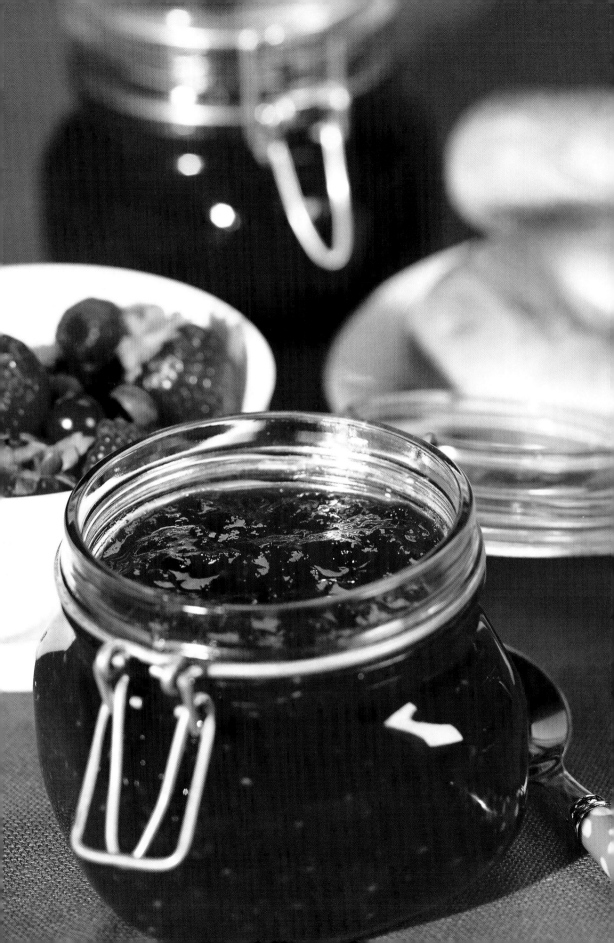

2. Brush bottom and sides of soufflé dish with some of the melted butter; sprinkle with enough brown sugar to coat bottom and sides. Put one-third of bread slices in bottom of dish; sprinkle with half of the fruit mixture. Drizzle with some of the remaining butter. Repeat with remaining bread, fruit mixture and butter, ending with a layer of bread.

3. In another bowl, beat eggs; add sugar, nutmeg, cinnamon, milk, cognac and vanilla. Pour slowly into soufflé dish, gently pressing to ensure bread has absorbed the custard. Let soak in refrigerator for 15 minutes. Cover with a piece of buttered foil, making sure dish is well sealed.

4. Set rack in the bottom of pressure cooker. Fold a two-foot (60 cm) long piece of foil several times to make a strip that will be used to remove dish. Center dish on midpoint of strip and fold the ends together to make a handle. Use strip to lower dish into the cooker. Pour in enough water to come halfway up sides of dish.

5. Lock the lid in place and bring cooker up to full pressure over high heat. Reduce heat to medium-low, just to maintain even pressure, and cook for 45 minutes. Remove from heat and release pressure quickly. Using foil handle, lift dish out of cooker onto cooling rack. Remove foil lid. The pudding should be set and a toothpick inserted in the center should come out clean. If not, seal with foil and return to cooker. Bring up to full pressure and cook for 2 minutes longer. Remove from heat and release pressure quickly. When pudding is cooked, remove foil lid. Serve warm or let cool on rack. (Cover and refrigerate until chilled, if desired.)

6. Meanwhile, make the Brandy Cream Sauce: In the top of a double boiler, combine cream, milk and vanilla; bring just to a simmer. In a bowl whisk together sugar, salt and egg yolks; slowly whisk in some of the hot cream mixture. Whisk egg mixture gradually back into double boiler and cook over medium heat, stirring constantly, until thick. Let cool in refrigerator. Stir in brandy.

7. Reheat pudding in microwave or steamer. Slice and serve with the brandy sauce.

Poached Winter Fruit Compote

Serves 4 to 6

Serve this light and healthy fruit dessert with a dollop of lemon yogurt or *crème fraîche*. It also makes a nice treat for brunch or spooned over pound cake.

Crème fraîche is made by combining 2 cups (500 mL) whipping (35%) cream with 1/2 cup (125 mL) sour cream, and letting the mixture stand at room temperature for 12 to 24 hours to thicken. Refrigerate the *crème fraîche* up to 2 weeks.

3	firm cooking apples (such as Northern Spy or Rome Beauty)	3
3	firm, underripe pears (Bosc variety holds its shape best; or use Bartlett)	3
1	seedless orange	1
1 cup	apple juice	250 mL
1 cup	dry white wine	250 mL
2 tbsp	buckwheat honey (or other dark honey)	25 mL
1	cinnamon stick	1
1/4 tsp	ground nutmeg	1 mL
	Zest of 1 lemon, minced	
1/2 cup	dried cranberries *or* dried cherries	125 mL
1/2 cup	vanilla *or* lemon yogurt	125 mL
	Cinnamon for dusting	

1. Peel and core apples and pears; cut into wedges. Set aside. Remove zest from orange; set aside. Cut peel from orange and cut out segments. Cover and refrigerate until serving.

2. In a pressure cooker, combine apple juice, wine, honey, cinnamon stick and nutmeg; bring to a boil. Reduce heat and simmer for 1 minute. Add apples, pears, orange zest and lemon zest.

3. Lock the lid in place and bring cooker up to full pressure over high heat. Reduce heat to medium-low, just to maintain even pressure, and cook for 1 minute. Remove from heat and release pressure quickly.

4. Using a slotted spoon, transfer fruit to a bowl. Bring remaining syrup to a boil; continue boiling to reduce and thicken. Pour syrup over the fruit and stir in dried cranberries. Cover and refrigerate overnight. Stir in orange segments. Serve in individual bowls, each with a dollop of yogurt or *crème fraîche* (see note, at left) and a dusting of cinnamon.

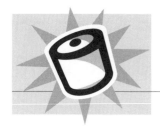

Creamy Rice Pudding with Sun-Dried Cranberries

1 cup	Arborio or other short-grain rice	250 mL
2 tbsp	butter	25 mL
2 cups	water	500 mL
1	can (14 oz [385 or 398 mL]) 2 % evaporated milk	1
1/2 tsp	ground cinnamon	2 mL
1/4 tsp	freshly grated nutmeg	1 mL
1/2 cup	dried cranberries, dried cherries or raisins	125 mL
1/2 cup	low-fat sweetened condensed milk	125 mL
1 tsp	vanilla extract	5 mL

Serves 4 to 6

The pressure cooker is ideal for making risotto. And here we have a sweet version of the rice dish which, combined with milk and dried fruit, makes a deliciously comforting dessert.

Don't worry if the pudding looks soupy when you remove the lid; the rice will absorb more liquid as it cools.

1. In a pressure cooker, melt butter over medium heat. Stir in rice, coating the grains with butter. Stir in water, evaporated milk, cinnamon and nutmeg; bring mixture to a boil over medium heat, stirring to make sure the milk doesn't burn.

2. Lock the lid in place and bring cooker up to full pressure over medium-high heat. Reduce heat to medium-low, just to maintain even pressure, and cook for 6 to 7 minutes. Remove cooker from heat and allow pressure to drop naturally for about 7 minutes. Remove lid.

3. Stir in dried cranberries, condensed milk and vanilla. Let stand, covered (do not lock), for 5 minutes. Spoon pudding into individual dishes and serve warm, or cover with plastic and chill to serve cold.

Steamy Chocolate Pudding with Vanilla Crème Anglaise

4-CUP (1 L) PUDDING MOLD, SOUFFLÉ DISH *OR* BUNDT PAN, BUTTERED AND FLOURED (USE SMALLER SIZE IF NECESSARY TO FIT INSIDE PRESSURE COOKER)

RACK OR TRIVET TO FIT BOTTOM OF PRESSURE COOKER

Serves 6

This decadent chocolate pudding is like a big, dense, steamy brownie. Serve it warm out of the pressure cooker in a pool of heavenly vanilla crème anglaise or with a scoop of frozen vanilla yogurt for a wonderful temperature contrast.

To ensure that puddings have a cake-like texture, it's best to have a dual-pressure machine. The lower pressure setting (8 psi) requires more cooking time, but this allows the puddings to rise. Under high pressure, steamed puddings remain very dense. And while these compacted desserts are still quite delicious, I prefer the lighter results you get using the low-pressure setting.

3 oz	bittersweet chocolate, chopped	75 g
1/2 cup	butter, softened	125 mL
3/4 cup	granulated sugar	175 mL
2	eggs, separated	2
1 tsp	vanilla extract	5 mL
1 cup	all-purpose flour	250 mL
1 tsp	baking powder	5 mL
1 tsp	baking soda	5 mL
Pinch	salt	Pinch
2/3 cup	milk	150 mL
2 cups	water for steaming	500 mL

VANILLA CRÈME ANGLAISE

3/4 cup	confectioner's (icing) sugar	175 mL
1 tsp	cornstarch	5 mL
2	egg yolks	2
2 tbsp	unsalted butter, melted	25 mL
1 cup	milk	250 mL
2 tsp	vanilla extract (or other flavoring, such as rum or coffee liqueur)	10 mL
1 cup	whipping (35%) cream, whipped	250 mL

1. In a heatproof bowl, set over hot (not boiling) water, melt chocolate. Let cool. In a bowl with an electric mixer, beat butter with sugar until fluffy. Beat in egg yolks and vanilla.

2. In a separate bowl, combine flour, baking powder, baking soda and salt. On low speed, beat dry ingredients into butter mixture alternately with milk, making three additions of flour and two of milk. Beat in chocolate.

3. In another bowl, beat egg whites until stiff peaks form. Gently fold into chocolate mixture. Pour into prepared mold. Cover with lid or a piece of foil.

4. Set rack in bottom of pressure cooker. Pour in water. Fold a two-foot (60 cm) long piece of foil several times to make a strip that will be used to remove mold. Center mold on midpoint of strip and fold the ends together to make a handle. Use strip to lower mold into the cooker.

5. Lock the lid in place and bring cooker up to low pressure over high heat. Reduce heat to medium-low, just to maintain even pressure, and cook for 40 minutes (or cook at full pressure for 20 minutes). Remove from heat and allow pressure to drop naturally for 8 to 10 minutes. Release any remaining pressure quickly. Using foil handle, lift the mold out of cooker onto cooling rack. Remove foil lid. Let cool for 30 minutes on rack. Run a sharp knife around the edge of pudding to loosen and invert onto a plate to cool completely.

6. VANILLA CRÈME ANGLAISE: In a bowl whisk together sugar, cornstarch, egg yolk and butter. In a double boiler, heat milk until steaming. Whisk a little of the hot milk into the sugar mixture. Gradually whisk back into the double boiler. Cook over simmering water, whisking constantly, until thick enough to coat a spoon. (Do not let the sauce boil or it will curdle.) Remove from heat and stir in vanilla. Whisk for 5 minutes to cool. Fold whipped cream into custard. Keep chilled in refrigerator. To serve, slice pudding and present in a pool of crème anglaise, or with frozen vanilla yogurt on the side.

Cool Lemon Custard with Fresh Berry Compote

Serves 6

TIP

You can also make this pudding in a straight-sided 5-cup (1.25 L) soufflé dish. Cook under pressure for 20 minutes if using a larger mold.

1/2 cup	granulated sugar	125 mL
1 tbsp	cornstarch	15 mL
2 1/2 cups	milk *or* cream	625 mL
2	eggs	2
2	egg yolks	2
	Finely grated zest of 1 lemon	
1/4 cup	fresh lemon juice	50 mL
2 cups	water for steaming	500 mL
	Confectioner's (icing) sugar (optional)	

BERRY COMPOTE

1/2 cup	granulated sugar	125 mL
1/4 cup	water	50 mL
1 cup	mixed berries (such as blueberries, Saskatoons, cranberries, raspberries)	250 mL
2 tbsp	brandy or orange brandy	25 mL

1. In a bowl whisk together sugar, cornstarch, milk, eggs, egg yolks, lemon zest and lemon juice. Pour into custard cups. Cover each with foil, making sure cups are well sealed.

2. Set rack in bottom of cooker. Pour in water. Place custard cups on rack, stacking if necessary. Lock the lid in place and bring cooker up to full pressure over high heat. Reduce heat to medium-low, just to maintain even pressure, and cook for 12 minutes. Remove from heat and release pressure quickly. Carefully lift cups out and place on a wire rack. Remove foil. Let cool to room temperature. Chill overnight in the refrigerator.

3. BERRY COMPOTE: In a saucepan combine sugar and water; bring to a boil over medium heat. Add berries and cook until they begin to break down and release their juices. Most of the berries should remain whole. Remove from heat, stir in brandy and chill.

4. To serve, run a sharp knife around edge of puddings and invert onto individual dessert plates. Top with berry compote. Dust with confectioner's sugar, if desired.

Steamed Lemon Poppyseed Cake

Serves 8

You won't find a moister poppyseed cake than this one. The recipe is based on Sue Spicer's favorite family cake and one of my quick coffee cake glazes.

Like a rich pound cake, this dessert is even better if you wrap it well and store it for a day or two before serving.

You'll need to use a low pressure setting and a longer cooking time to get this cake to rise properly.

4-CUP (1 L) SOUFFLÉ DISH OR BUNDT PAN, GREASED AND FLOURED
RACK OR TRIVET TO FIT BOTTOM OF PRESSURE COOKER

1/2 cup	butter, softened	125 mL
1 cup	granulated sugar	250 mL
2	eggs, separated	2
1 tsp	vanilla extract	5 mL
	Zest of 2 lemons, divided	
	Juice of 2 lemons, divided	
1 1/4 cup	all-purpose flour	300 mL
1 tsp	baking soda	5 mL
1 tsp	baking powder	5 mL
1/2 tsp	salt	2 mL
2/3 cup	milk	175 mL
1/3 cup	poppyseeds	75 mL
2 cups	water for steaming	500 mL

GLAZE

1/2 cup	confectioner's (icing) sugar	125 mL

1. In a bowl with an electric mixer, beat butter with sugar until light and fluffy. Beat in egg yolks and vanilla. Beat in half of the lemon zest and lemon juice.

2. In a separate bowl, combine flour, baking soda, baking powder and salt. Beat dry ingredients into butter-sugar mixture, alternating with the milk, making three additions of dry and two of milk. Fold in poppyseeds.

3. In another bowl, beat egg whites until stiff. Gently fold into batter until just combined. Pour into prepared dish. Cover with a piece of foil, making sure dish is well sealed.

4. Set rack in bottom of cooker. Pour in water. Fold a two-foot (60 cm) long piece of foil several times to make a strip that will be used to remove dish. Center dish on midpoint of strip and fold the ends together to make a handle. Use strip to lower dish into the cooker.

5. Lock the lid in place and bring cooker up to low pressure over high heat. Reduce heat to medium-low, just to maintain even pressure, and cook for 40 minutes (or cook at full pressure for 20 minutes). Remove from heat and allow pressure to drop naturally. Using foil handle, lift dish out of cooker onto cooling rack. Remove foil lid. Let cool completely.

6. GLAZE: Whisk remaining lemon zest and lemon juice together with confectioner's sugar. To serve, turn the cake out onto a serving platter and drizzle with glaze.

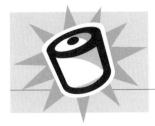

Poached Pears in Spiced Red Wine

Serves 6

You can serve this easy-but-elegant fall dessert warm from the pan or chilled with a dollop of lemon yogurt. Be sure to use slightly underripe pears and leave them whole, with stems intact, for a dramatic presentation.

TIP

Choose a nice light red wine for this recipe, such as Beaujolais, Grenache, Pinot Noir or a young Chianti.

6	firm, slightly underripe pears (preferably Bosc or Comice)	6
1	lemon	1
1/2 cup	granulated sugar	125 mL
3	whole cloves	3
1	cinnamon stick	1
2 cups	light red wine	500 mL
	Lemon yogurt as accompaniment	
	Mint leaves for garnish	

1. Peel pears and, using an apple corer or small melon baller, remove cores from bottoms, leaving stems intact and pears whole. Cut a thin slice from the bottom of each pear so they will stand upright. Using a vegetable peeler, remove zest from lemon in large strips. Reserve lemon for another use.

2. In a pressure cooker, combine lemon zest, sugar, cloves, cinnamon and wine; cook over medium heat until sugar is dissolved. Stand pears in pot.

3. Lock the lid in place and bring cooker up to full pressure over high heat. Reduce heat to medium-low, just to maintain even pressure, and cook for 4 minutes. Remove from heat and release pressure quickly.

4. Remove the lid and let pears cool in their liquid. With a slotted spoon, carefully transfer pears to a shallow dish. Boil poaching liquid over high heat until reduced, glossy and syrupy. Spoon syrup over pears and cool slightly, or chill them overnight.

5. Serve pears whole (or sliced lengthwise up to the stem and fanned) on individual dessert plates with some of the syrup drizzled over them. If served cold, garnish with a dollop of lemon yogurt and a mint leaf.

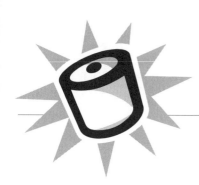

Stocks, Sauces & Condiments

Tips for Making Stocks

With a pressure cooker, you can make fast and healthy stocks from scratch in less than an hour.

Instead of discarding vegetable peelings, meat and poultry trimmings, fish bones, turkey carcasses and other kitchen scraps, freeze them in plastic bags until you're ready to make the stock.

You can use almost any vegetable in a stock, but avoid strong-tasting members of the cabbage family, turnips and leafy greens. Unless you're making borscht, avoid red beets, which will turn your stock a deep magenta color. If you use vegetable peelings for stock, make sure that the vegetables are well scrubbed.

Browning vegetables and meats before simmering will yield a darker, richer-tasting stock. If you're pressed for time – or simply want a lighter stock – simply skip the browning step.

It's usually best to make your stocks without salt, then season the final dish to taste when it's done.

Refrigerate stocks and skim off any congealed fat before using them. Stocks can be refrigerated for up to 3 days or frozen for up to 6 months. Or you can reduce a stock to one-quarter of its volume and freeze it in ice cube trays, then reconstitute them for use in recipes.

Vegetable Stock

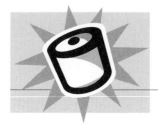

*Makes 6 to 8 cups
(1.5 to 2 L)*

TIP

You can also use clean peelings from carrots and parsnips in this vegetarian stock.

2 tbsp	butter *or* olive oil	25 mL
4	cloves garlic, peeled	4
3	sprigs parsley	3
2	carrots, scrubbed and chopped	2
2	stalks celery, coarsely chopped	2
1	large onion, quartered	1
1	parsnip, scrubbed and chopped	1
1	tomato, chopped	1
1	bay leaf	1
1	sprig thyme	1
8 cups	water	2 L

1. In a pressure cooker, heat butter over medium heat. Add garlic, parsley, carrots, celery, onion, parsnip, tomato, bay leaf and thyme; sauté for 10 minutes or until softened. Pour in water.

2. Lock the lid in place and bring cooker up to full pressure over high heat. Reduce heat to medium-low, just to maintain even pressure, and cook for 15 minutes. Remove from heat and allow pressure to drop naturally.

3. Strain stock through a fine mesh sieve, pressing on the solids to release all of their liquid. Discard the solids.

Brown Stock

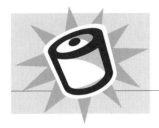

*Makes 5 to 6 cups
(1.25 to 1.5 mL)*

You can use this recipe to make stock from beef and/or pork bones, game trimmings, lamb or duck. For lamb stock, augment with garlic. Game stock is improved by the addition of several juniper berries and dried mushrooms. A tart apple adds a nice sweetness to duck broth.

TIP

To make a demiglace from this stock, simmer until reduced to 1 cup (250 mL), then freeze in ice cube trays. Transfer frozen cubes to a zippered freezer bag and use as a base for sauces or soups.

If you are making more than one batch of stock in the pressure cooker, speed up the process by combining bones and oil in a shallow roasting pan and roast in a 400° F (200° C) oven for 1 hour. Drain off fat and transfer to cooker. Proceed with adding vegetables.

The darker the bones, the richer and more deeply colored your final stock will be.

2 tbsp	vegetable oil	25 mL
2 lbs	beef, veal and/or pork bones, cut into 2-inch (5 cm) pieces	1 kg
1 cup	chopped mixed vegetables or trimmings (onion, carrot, celery, leek, parsnip)	250 mL
1	plum tomato, seeded and chopped	1
1 tsp	whole black peppercorns	5 mL
6 cups	cold water	1.5 L
1 cup	dry red wine	250 mL
	Fresh herbs (such as thyme, parsley, rosemary, etc.)	

1. In a pressure cooker, heat oil over medium-high heat. Add bones in batches and cook until browned. Drain any excess fat. Return bones to cooker and add vegetables; sauté, until vegetables start to brown. Add tomato, peppercorns, water, wine and herbs.

2. Lock the lid in place and bring cooker up to full pressure over high heat. Reduce heat to medium-low, just to maintain even pressure, and cook for 30 minutes. Remove from heat and allow pressure to drop naturally.

3. Strain stock through a cheesecloth-lined fine mesh sieve. Discard remaining solids. Let cool, cover and refrigerate overnight. Remove any excess fat that has solidified on top before using the stock or freezing it.

Chicken or Turkey Stock

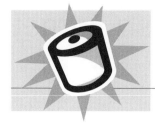

Makes about 8 cups (2 L)

This stock is useful for many dishes – including the famously comforting chicken soup, the perfect antidote to a winter cold.

Don't throw out the bones after your holiday turkey is picked clean – the carcass is perfect for making flavorful turkey broth.

When the stock is cooked, you can salvage any meat from the chicken or turkey and add it, along with some small egg noodles, to the broth and boil until tender. Look for tiny imported egg noodles in European delis – they make the best chicken soup.

2 to 3 lbs	chicken bones, a small stewing hen *or* 1 turkey carcass	1 to 1.5 kg
5	whole peppercorns	5
5	sprigs parsley	5
2	stalks celery	2
2	carrots, scrubbed	2
1	parsnip, scrubbed	1
1	large onion, quartered	1
1	sprig fresh thyme	1
1	bay leaf	1
8 to 12 cups	cold water	2 to 3 L

1. In a pressure cooker, combine chicken, peppercorns, parsley, celery, carrots, parsnip, onion, thyme and bay leaf. Pour in as much water as necessary to reach maximum fill level advised by the manufacturer.

2. Lock the lid in place and bring cooker up to full pressure over high heat. Reduce heat to medium-low, just to maintain even pressure, and cook for 20 to 30 minutes (depending on the amount of chicken used). Remove from heat and allow pressure to drop naturally.

3. Strain stock through a cheesecloth-lined fine mesh sieve, pressing on the solids to release all of their liquid. Discard remaining solids.

4. Allow stock to cool, then cover and refrigerate overnight. Remove any excess fat that has solidified on top before using the stock or freezing it.

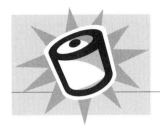

Fish Fumet

*Makes 6 to 8 cups
(1.5 to 2 L)*

Good fish stock is the basis for many soups and chowders. Ask your fishmonger for fish heads and bones (both are good for stock), or save your own fish scraps in the freezer. Shrimp and lobster shells also make good fish stock. Be sure to use non-fatty fish, such as halibut, sole and turbot; salmon scraps are not good for stock.

1 lb	fish bones and trimmings	500 g
5	black peppercorns	5
2	stalks celery, cut into chunks	2
1	carrot, quartered	1
1	small onion, halved	1
1	bay leaf	1
1	sprig thyme	1
1	sprig parsley	1
1/2 tsp	fennel seed	2 mL
1/2 cup	dry white wine	125 mL
8 cups	cold water (approximate)	2 L

1. In a pressure cooker, combine fish bones and trimmings, peppercorns, celery, carrot, onion, bay leaf, thyme, parsley, fennel seed and wine. Pour in as much water as necessary to reach maximum fill level advised by the manufacturer. Bring to a boil and skim off any foam that rises to the surface.

2. Lock the lid in place and bring cooker up to full pressure over high heat. Reduce heat to medium-low, just to maintain even pressure, and cook for 15 minutes. Remove cooker from heat and allow pressure to drop naturally.

3. Strain stock through a fine-mesh sieve, pressing on the solids to release all of their liquid. Discard remaining solids. Cool stock and refrigerate or freeze for future use.

Basic Tomato and Vegetable Sauce for Pasta

Makes 4 to 5 cups (1 to 1.25 L)

TIP

This versatile pasta sauce will keep 3 days in the refrigerator or up to 3 months in the freezer.

1/4 cup	olive oil	50 mL
1 cup	chopped onions	250 mL
3	cloves garlic, minced	3
1	small zucchini, chopped	1
1	large carrot, chopped	1
1 cup	chopped eggplant	250 mL
1/2 cup	chopped red or yellow bell peppers	125 mL
1/2 cup	chopped fresh mushrooms	125 mL
1	can (28 oz [796 mL]) crushed tomatoes	1
1 tsp	dried oregano	5 mL
1 tsp	dried basil	5 mL
1/4 cup	tomato paste	50 mL
1 tsp	granulated sugar	5 mL
1/4 tsp	red pepper flakes	1 mL
	Salt and freshly ground black pepper to taste	

1. In a pressure cooker, heat oil over medium-high heat. Add garlic and onion; sauté until they start to brown. Stir in zucchini, carrot, eggplant, peppers and mushrooms; cook for 5 minutes longer. Add tomatoes, oregano and basil.

2. Lock the lid in place and bring cooker up to full pressure over high heat. Reduce heat to medium-low, just to maintain even pressure, and cook for 8 minutes. Remove from heat and allow pressure to drop naturally.

3. Stir in tomato paste. (If desired, purée some or all of the sauce with an immersion blender or in a food processor.) Stir in sugar and red pepper flakes. Season to taste with salt and pepper.

My Favorite Barbecue Sauce

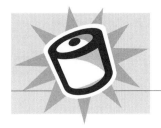

Makes 3 1/2 cups
(875 mL)

There's nothing to beat a flavorful, homemade barbecue sauce. This one is a little sweet and spicy, perfect for brushing on burgers. If you like your barbecue bastes even spicier, torque up this recipe with some hot sauce.

3	cloves garlic, minced	3
1	chipotle chili in adobo, chopped *or* 1 jalapeño pepper, chopped and 1 tsp (5 mL) liquid smoke	1
1	large onion, minced	1
1/2 cup	packed brown sugar	125 mL
1 tbsp	dried basil	15 mL
1 tbsp	chili powder	15 mL
1 tsp	ground cumin	5 mL
1 cup	dark beer	250 mL
1 cup	ketchup	250 mL
1/2 cup	canned beef broth, undiluted	125 mL
2 tbsp	Dijon mustard	25 mL
1 tbsp	Worcestershire sauce	15 mL
	Salt and freshly ground black pepper to taste	

1. In a pressure cooker, combine garlic, chipotle, onion, sugar, chili powder, basil, cumin, beer, ketchup, broth, mustard and Worcestershire; stir until sugar is dissolved.

2. Lock the lid in place and bring cooker up to full pressure over high heat. Reduce heat to medium-low, just to maintain even pressure, and cook for 6 minutes. Remove from heat and release pressure quickly.

3. Season to taste with salt and pepper. Simmer, uncovered, over medium heat for about 10 minutes or until reduced and thickened to desired consistency. For a smooth sauce, purée with an immersion blender or in a food processor. Pour the sauce into a clean jar and refrigerate for up to 1 week.

Cowboy Ranchero Sauce

*Makes 4 to 5 cups
(1 to 1.25 L)*

Use this southwestern vegetarian sauce over pasta, spooned over a meatloaf or enchiladas before baking, or as a braising sauce for chicken.

16	plum tomatoes (about 4 lbs [2 kg]), cored and halved	16
12	serrano chilies, seeded and halved	12
6	cloves garlic, peeled	6
2	large sweet onions, chopped	2
1 cup	beer	250 mL
2 tbsp	honey (or to taste)	25 mL
	Salt to taste	
1 cup	chopped cilantro leaves	250 mL

1. In a pressure cooker, combine tomatoes, chilies, garlic, onions and beer. Lock the lid in place and bring cooker up to full pressure over high heat. Reduce heat to medium-low, just to maintain even pressure, and cook for 7 minutes. Remove from heat and release pressure quickly.

2. Strain sauce through a sieve, reserving the liquid. Transfer solids to a food processor and purée until smooth. Return to cooker and add honey to taste. Stir in enough of the reserved cooking liquid to create a smooth sauce. Season to taste with salt. Stir in cilantro just before serving.

Italian Sausage and Tomato Ragu Sauce

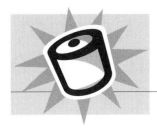

Makes 5 cups (1.25 L)

Start with a good-quality sweet or spicy Italian sausage and you have an instantly flavorful meat sauce to serve over pasta or use in lasagna. This basic meat sauce is ideal for any great Italian-style supper.

TIP

For a Greek-style sauce, use 1/2 tsp (2 mL) cinnamon instead of pesto or basil to finish the sauce.

Instead of simmering the sauce to thicken, mash together 1 to 2 tbsp (15 to 25 mL) softened butter with 1 to 2 tbsp (15 to 25 mL) all-purpose flour and whisk into sauce; cook, stirring, for about 5 minutes or until thickened.

1 tbsp	olive oil	15 mL
1 lb	sweet or spicy Italian sausage, casings removed, meat crumbled	500 g
8 oz	lean ground beef	250 g
4	cloves garlic, minced	4
2	onions, finely chopped	2
1	red or yellow bell pepper, chopped	1
1 cup	finely chopped mushrooms	250 mL
1	carrot, shredded	1
2 1/2 tsp	dried oregano	12 mL
1/2 tsp	fennel seed	2 mL
1	bay leaf	1
1 tsp	granulated sugar	5 mL
2 cups	canned plum tomatoes, crushed or puréed in blender	500 mL
2 cups	tomato juice	500 mL
1/2 cup	red wine	125 mL
1/4 cup	tomato paste	50 mL
1 tbsp	basil pesto *or* chopped basil	15 mL
	Salt and freshly ground black pepper to taste	

1. In a pressure cooker, heat oil over medium heat. Add sausage and ground beef; cook, breaking up meat with a spoon, until no longer pink.
2. Add garlic, onions, red pepper, and mushrooms; sauté for 5 minutes. Stir in carrot, oregano and fennel; cook for 1 minute longer. Stir in bay leaf, sugar, tomatoes, tomato juice, wine and tomato paste.
3. Lock the lid in place and bring cooker up to full pressure over high heat. Reduce heat to medium-low, just to maintain even pressure, and cook for 20 minutes. Remove from heat and release pressure quickly.
4. Simmer, uncovered, to reduce slightly. Stir in pesto and season to taste with salt and pepper. Store in the refrigerator for 2 days or freeze for up to 1 month.

Tips for Making Jams and Chutneys

The pressure cooker speeds up the jam-making process in two ways: It quickly softens and cooks fruit to a pulpy purée; and it infuses the mixture with the flavors of added whole spices. Cooking under pressure can reduce preparation time by 50 to 70 percent in most recipes.

The main rule to keep in mind when making jams and chutneys is never to overfill the pressure cooker. If you are adapting a traditional preserve recipe for pressure cooking, it's always best to be cautious and never fill the cooker more than half full.

Start by preparing fruit preserves in the traditional way – allowing the fruit and sugar to sit for about 1 hour in the pressure cooker, so that the fruits' natural juices are released. Then bring fruit and sugar to a boil, stirring, before locking the lid in place and bringing the cooker up to pressure.

For jams that must reach an acceptable gel point, cook the fruit and sugar together for up to 8 minutes under pressure, then allow pressure to drop naturally and rapidly boil the mixture for an additional 2 to 5 minutes until a bit spooned on an ice-cold plate, chilled in the freezer, sets up and congeals. You should start checking the gel after about 2 to 3 minutes of cooking, then continue to boil the jam until it is set to your liking. Some mixtures may take up to 20 minutes of cooking if you are looking for a very stiff result, but will reach a softer gel point much sooner. It's up to you.

The recipes in this chapter are for small batches of preserves, which are intended to be refrigerated and served within 3 days, or frozen for up to 1 month, although all can be canned conventionally for longer storage.

For complete instructions on canning jams and chutneys for longer room-temperature storage, consult a specialty book like the *Bernardin Guide to Home Preserving*, published by Bernardin Canada, or *Clearly Delicious*, by Elisabeth Lambert Ortiz (Macmillan Canada).

Strawberry Jam

Makes 4 cups (1 L)

The pressure cooker makes this smooth-textured jam so quickly, all of the intense straw-berry color is preserved. If you have 6-litre machine, you can easily double the recipe.

4 cups	hulled strawberries, halved	1 L
3 cups	granulated sugar	750 mL
	Juice of 1 lemon	

1. In a pressure cooker, combine strawberries and sugar. Let stand for 30 to 60 minutes, until juicy. Using a potato masher, mash fruit, making sure all of the sugar is dissolved. Stir in lemon juice; bring to a boil.

2. Lock the lid in place and bring cooker up to full pressure over high heat. Reduce heat to medium-low, just to maintain even pressure, and cook for 7 minutes. Remove cooker from heat and allow pressure to drop naturally.

3. Remove the lid. Bring to a rapid boil over high heat; boil, uncovered, for about 3 minutes, or just until jam reaches the gel stage (when a bit spooned onto an ice-cold plate sets up and congeals; see page 181 for details). Skim off any foam and ladle into hot sterilized jars, leaving 1/2 inch (1 cm) head space. Seal jars. Cool and refrigerate up to 1 week, freeze for up to 1 month, or process for shelf storage.

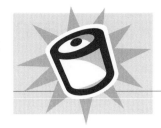

Fresh Apricot Jam

*Makes 6 to 7 cups
(1.5 to 1.75 L)*

This recipe makes a very smooth, softly-set apricot jam, perfect for glazing fruit tarts or other desserts. If you prefer a chunkier jam, only purée a portion of the fresh apricots with the orange flesh in the food processor.

6 cups	apricots, halved	1.5 L
1	large navel orange, peeled	1
1/2 cup	water *or* apple juice	125 mL
6 cups	granulated sugar	1.5 L

1. In a food processor, chop apricots and orange with water, in batches if necessary. Pour into a pressure cooker. Stir in sugar and let stand for 30 minutes. Bring to a boil, stirring until sugar is dissolved.

2. Lock the lid in place and bring cooker up to full pressure over high heat. Reduce heat to medium-low, just to maintain even pressure, and cook for 8 minutes. Remove from heat and allow pressure to drop naturally.

3. Remove the lid. Bring to a rapid boil over high heat; boil, uncovered, for about 3 minutes, or just until jam reaches the gel stage (when a bit spooned onto an ice-cold plate sets up and congeals; see page 181 for details). Skim off any foam and ladle into hot sterilized jars, leaving 1/2 inch (1 cm) head space. Seal jars. Cool and refrigerate up to 1 week, freeze for up to 1 month, or process for shelf storage.

Spiced Dried Apricot Jam

Makes about 7 cups (1.75 L)

The aromatic spices in this jam give it a lovely flavor and aroma. While it's delicious on scones for breakfast, it also makes a wonderful accompaniment to pork roast or pâté.

TIP

Look for star anise (a large star-shaped pod) and cardamom seeds at Asian or Indian grocery stores.

The dried fruit in this recipe results in a very firm jam; for a softer set, add more water.

4 cups	dried apricots, coarsely chopped	1 L
2 cups	water	500 mL
6	black peppercorns	6
5	cardamom pods	5
2	cinnamon sticks	2
2	star anise *or* 1 tsp (5 mL) anise or fennel seed	2
	Juice of 2 lemons	
4 cups	granulated sugar	1 L

1. In a bowl combine the apricots and water. Cover and let soak for 24 hours.

2. In a square of cheesecloth, wrap peppercorns, cardamom pods, cinnamon sticks and star anise; tie into a bag with kitchen string. (Or place ingredients in a tea ball.)

3. Add apricots and spice bag to pressure cooker. Stir in lemon juice. Lock the lid in place and bring cooker up to full pressure over high heat. Reduce heat to medium-low, just to maintain even pressure, and cook for 10 minutes. Remove from heat and allow pressure to drop naturally.

3. Discard spice bag. Stir in sugar. Bring to a rapid boil over high heat; boil, uncovered, for about 3 to 4 minutes, until gel point is reached (when a bit spooned onto an ice-cold plate sets up and congeals; see page 181 for details). Skim off any foam and ladle into hot sterilized jars, leaving 1/2 inch (1 cm) head space. Seal jars. Cool and refrigerate up to 1 week, freeze for up to 1 month, or process for shelf storage.

Mixed Berry and Red Fruit Jam

Makes 6 cups (1.5 mL)

Use fresh or frozen fruit for this rich, inky, mixed-berry jam. If you like, substitute chopped prunes or dark raisins for the black currants.

1 lb	cranberries	500 g
8 oz	raspberries	250 g
8 oz	blueberries	250 g
8 oz	strawberries, chopped	250 g
4 oz	rhubarb, chopped	125 g
4 oz	dried black currants	125 g
	Zest and juice of 1 lemon	
6 cups	granulated sugar	1.5 L

1. In a pressure cooker, combine cranberries, raspberries, blueberries, strawberries, rhubarb, black currants, lemon zest, lemon juice and sugar; let stand for 30 to 60 minutes, until juicy. Bring to a boil, adding up to 1/4 cup (50 mL) water if necessary to dissolve sugar.

2. Lock the lid in place and bring cooker up to full pressure over high heat. Reduce heat to medium-low, just to maintain even pressure, and cook for 10 minutes. Remove from heat and allow pressure to drop naturally.

3. Remove the lid. Boil jam rapidly for about 3 to 4 minutes, until gel point is reached (when a bit spooned onto an ice-cold plate sets up and congeals; see page 181 for details). Skim off any foam and ladle into hot sterilized jars, leaving 1/2 inch (1 cm) headspace. Seal jars. Cool and refrigerate up to 1 week, freeze for up to 1 month, or process for shelf storage.

Pear Mincemeat

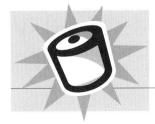

Makes 5 cups (1.25 L)

TIP

Use a heavy, covered canner or stock pot for processing preserves. If you don't have a proper canner (with a wire lifting insert) place a metal rack in the bottom of the pot. The canner or pot should be large enough so that when submerged, jars will be covered by about 1 inch (2 cm) of boiling water.

Seal filled jars with metal lids and rings, closing until just "finger tip" tight. Carefully lower jars into boiling water using a jar lifter until they are all submerged in a single layer. Cover the pan. When water returns to a full, rolling boil, start timing the processing. Lift processed jars from water and set on a folded towel on the counter to cool. When you hear the lids pop down as the preserves cool, you will know you have a proper seal.

2 1/2 lbs	pears, peeled, cored and chopped	1.25 kg
1	green apple, peeled, cored and chopped	1
	Zest and juice of 1 lemon	
	Zest and juice of 1 orange	
1 cup	golden raisins	250 mL
1/2 cup	dried cranberries or currants	125 mL
1/2 cup	packed brown sugar	125 mL
1 tsp	ground cinnamon	5 mL
1 tsp	ground nutmeg	5 mL
1/4 tsp	ground ginger	1 mL
Pinch	salt	Pinch
1/2 cup	chopped walnuts or pecans, toasted	125 mL
1/2 cup	cognac *or* pear brandy	125 mL

1. In a pressure cooker, combine pears, apple, lemon zest, lemon juice, orange zest, orange juice, raisins, cranberries, sugar, cinnamon, nutmeg, ginger and salt. Bring to a boil over medium heat.

2. Lock the lid in place and bring cooker up to full pressure over high heat. Reduce heat to medium-low, just to maintain even pressure, and cook for 10 minutes. Remove from heat and allow pressure to drop naturally.

3. Simmer, uncovered, for 10 minutes or until mixture is very thick. Stir in walnuts and cognac; cook for 5 minutes longer. Ladle into hot, sterilized jars, leaving 1/2 inch (1 cm) headspace. Seal jars. Cool and refrigerate, freeze, or process in a boiling water bath for shelf storage.

Index